# Preventive Health Measures
# for Lesbian
# and Bisexual Women

*Preventive Health Measures for Lesbian and Bisexual Women* has been co-published simultaneously as *Women & Health*, Volume 44, Number 2 2006.

D1606273

## Monographic Separates from *Women & Health*™

For additional information on these and other Haworth Press titles, including descriptions, tables of contents, reviews, and prices, use the QuickSearch catalog at http://www.HaworthPress.com.

*Preventive Health Measures for Lesbian and Bisexual Women,* edited by Shelly Kerr, PhD, and Robin Mathy, MA, MSc, MSW (Vol. 44, No. 2, 2006). *Examination of the latest research and preventative health measures for lesbian and bisexual women.*

*Women's Health: New Frontiers in Advocacy & Social Justice Research,* edited by Elizabeth Cartwright, PhD, and Pascale Allotey, PhD (Vol. 43, No. 4, 2006). *Examines how researchers can become advocates when the marginalization of community groups affects access to the programs and services they need.*

*Teaching Gender, Teaching Women's Health: Case Studies in Medical and Health Science Education,* edited by Lenore Manderson, PhD, FASSA (Vol. 37, No. 4, 2003). *"VALUABLE to anyone involved in medical and health science education. . . . Provides much-needed insight." (Ursula K. Snyder, PhD, Editor/Program Director, Medscape Ob/Gyn & Women's Health, New York City)*

*Environmental, Policy and Cultural Factors Related to Physical Activity in a Diverse Sample of Women: The Women's Cardiovascular Health Network Project,* edited by Amy A. Eyler, PhD (Vol. 36, No. 2, 2002). *"INTERESTING AND UNIQUE. . . . A MUST-READ for anyone interested in designing, implementing, and evaluating physical activity interventions for underserved–and typically inactive–women." (Lynda Randsell, PhD, FACSM, Assistant Professor of Exercise & Sport Science, University of Utah-Salt Lake City)*

*Women's Health in Mainland Southeast Asia,* edited by Andrea Whittaker, PhD (Vol. 35, No. 4, 2002). *Shows how war, military regimes, industrialization, urbanization, and social upheaval have all affected the choices Southeast Asian women make about their health and health care.*

*Domestic Violence and Health Care: Policies and Prevention,* edited by Carolina Reyes, MD, William J. Rudman, PhD, and Calvin R. Hewitt, MBA (Vol. 35, No. 2/3, 2002). *Examines the role of health care in the struggle to combat domestic violence.*

*Women's Work, Health and Quality of Life,* edited by Afaf Ibrahim Meleis, PhD, FAAN (Vol. 33, No. 1/2, 2001). *"A FINE COLLECTION. . . . A useful supplement for courses on women and health. It is particularly helpful to have a collection that reports research on women in different countries. . . . Describes role overload, role strain, and stress that occurs when immigrants try to adjust to a new culture." (Eleanor Krassen Covan, PhD, Professor of Sociology, Director of Gerontology, University of North Carolina, Wilmington)*

*Welfare, Work and Well-Being,* edited by Mary Clare Lennon, PhD, MS (Vol. 32, No. 1/2 & No. 3, 2001). *Examines the relationship between social roles, economic circumstances, material hardship, and child well-being among low-income women.*

*Australian Women's Health: Innovations in Social Science and Community Research,* edited by Lenore Manderson, PhD (Vol. 28, No. 1, 1998). *Reflects a wider approach to women's health, which moves from maternity and fertility issues to question the impact of gender on all aspects of the disease experience.*

*Women, Drug Use and HIV Infection,* edited by Sally J. Stevens, PhD, Stephanie Tortu, PhD, and Susan L. Coyle, PhD (Vol. 27, No. 1/2, 1998). *"A much-needed resource of critical information about the largest initiative to date designed to prevent HIV among drug users and their sexual partners." (Robert E. Booth, PhD, Associate Professor of Psychiatry, University of Colorado School of Medicine, Denver)*

*Women in the Later Years: Health, Social, and Cultural Perspectives,* edited by Lois Grau, PhD, RN, in collaboration with Ida Susser, PhD (Vol. 14, No. 3/4, 1989). *"An excellent overview of the pertinent social, political, and personal issues of this long-ignored group." (News for Women in Psychiatry)*

***Government Policy and Women's Health Care: The Swedish Alternative,*** edited by Gunnela Westlander, PhD, and Jeanne Mager Stellman, PhD (Vol. 13, No. 3/4, 1988). *"An illuminating, comprehensive overview of Swedish women's health and their productive and reproductive roles." (Freda L. Paltiel, Senior Advisor, Status of Women, Health and Welfare Canada, Ottawa, Ontario, Canada)*

***Embryos, Ethics, and Women's Rights: Exploring the New Reproductive Technologies,*** edited by Elaine Hoffman Báruch, Amadeo F. D'Adamo, Jr., and Joni Seager (Vol. 13, No. 1/2, 1988). *"Groundbreaking . . . Reveals the myriad of perspectives from which the new technologies can be regarded. Particularly thought-provoking are discussions that link surrogacy to economic and class issues." (Publishers Weekly)*

***Women, Health, and Poverty (also published as Dealing with the Health Needs of Women in Poverty),*** edited by Cesar A. Perales and Lauren S. Young, EdD (Vol. 12, No. 3/4, 1988). *"Succeeds in alerting readers to many important issues. . . Should be useful to public policymakers, researchers, and others interested in understanding the health problems of poor women." (Contemporary Psychology)*

***Women and Cancer,*** edited by Steven D. Stellman, PhD (Vol. 11, No. 3/4, 1987). *"The contributors succeed in increasing the reader's awareness of cancer in women and in stimulating thought processes in reference to the need for further research." (Oncology Nursing Forum)*

***Health Needs of Women as They Age,*** edited by Sharon Golub, PhD, and Rita Jackaway Freedman, PhD (Vol. 10, No. 2/3, 1985). *"The contributors distill a great deal of general information on aging into an easily readable and understandable format . . . A useful primer." (The New England Journal of Medicine)*

***Health Care of the Female Adolescent,*** edited by Sharon Golub, PhD (Vol. 9, No. 2/3, 1985). *"An excellent collection of well-written and carefully selected articles designed to provide up-to-date information about the health problems of adolescent girls." (Journal of the American Medical Women's Association)*

***Lifting the Curse of Menstruation: A Feminist Appraisal of the Influence of Menstruation on Women's Lives,*** edited by Sharon Golub, PhD (Vol. 8, No. 2/3, 1983). *"Crammed with information and well-documented. Written in a professional style, each chapter is followed by extensive lists of notes and references." (Journal of Sex Education and Therapy)*

***Obstetrical Intervention and Technology in the 1980s,*** edited by Diony Young, BA (Vol. 7, No. 3/4, 1983). *"Every family physician and obstetrician in North America should read this book." (Canadian Family Physician)*

# Preventive Health Measures for Lesbian and Bisexual Women

Shelly Kerr, PhD
Robin Mathy, MA, MSc, MSW
Editors

*Preventive Health Measures for Lesbian and Bisexual Women* has been co-published simultaneously as *Women & Health*, Volume 44, Number 2 2006.

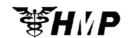

The Haworth Medical Press®
An Imprint of The Haworth Press, Inc.

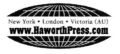

New York • London • Victoria (AU)
www.HaworthPress.com

Published by

The Haworth Medical Press®, 10 Alice Street, Binghamton, NY 13904-1580 USA

The Haworth Medical Press® is an imprint of The Haworth Press, Inc., 10 Alice Street, Binghamton, NY 13904-1580 USA.

*Preventive Health Measures for Lesbian and Bisexual Women* has been co-published simultaneously as *Women & Health*, Volume 44, Number 2 2006.

The development, preparation, and publication of this work has been undertaken with great care. However, the publisher, employees, editors, and agents of The Haworth Press and all imprints of The Haworth Press, Inc., including The Haworth Medical Press® and Pharmaceutical Products Press®, are not responsible for any errors contained herein or for consequences that may ensue from use of materials or information contained in this work. With regard to case studies, identities and circumstances of individuals discussed herein have been changed to protect confidentiality. Any resemblance to actual persons, living or dead, is entirely coincidental.

The Haworth Press is committed to the dissemination of ideas and information according to the highest standards of intellectual freedom and the free exchange of ideas. Statements made and opinions expressed in this publication do not necessarily reflect the views of the Publisher, Directors, management, or staff of The Haworth Press, Inc., or an endorsement by them.

### Library of Congress Cataloging-in-Publication Data

Preventive health measures for lesbian and bisexual women / Shelly Kerr, Robin Mathy, editors.
    p. ; cm.
    "Co-published simultaneously as women & health, volume 44, number 2."
    Includes bibliographical references and index.
    ISBN-13: 978-0-7890-3332-1 (hard cover : alk. paper)
    ISBN-10: 0-7890-3332-1 (hard cover : alk. paper)
    ISBN-13: 978-0-7890-3333-8 (soft cover : alk. paper)
    ISBN-10: 0-7890-3333-X (soft cover : alk. paper)
    1. Lesbians–Health and hygiene. 2. Lesbians–Diseases–Prevention. 3. Bisexual women–Health and hygiene. 4. Bisexual women–Diseases–Prevention. 5. Breast–Cancer–Prevention. I. Kerr, Shelly K. II. Mathy, Robin M.
    [DNLM: 1. Breast Neoplasms–prevention & control. 2. Bisexuality–psychology. 3. Evaluation Studies. 4. Health Behavior. 5. Homosexuality, Female–psychology. 6. Professional-Patient Relations. W1 WO478 v.44 no. 2 2006 / WP 870 P944 2006]
RA564.87.P74 2006
613.086'64–dc22

                                       2006029472

**The HAWORTH PRESS Inc.**

# Abstracting, Indexing & Outward Linking

PRINT *and* ELECTRONIC BOOKS & JOURNALS

This section provides you with a list of major indexing & abstracting services and other tools for bibliographic access. That is to say, each service began covering this periodical during the the year noted in the right column. Most Websites which are listed below have indicated that they will either post, disseminate, compile, archive, cite or alert their own Website users with research-based content from this work. (This list is as current as the copyright date of this publication.)

(continued)

(continued)

(continued)

(continued)

(continued)

# Bibliographic Access

- ***Magazines for Libraries (Katz)***

- ***Ulrich's Periodicals Directory: International Periodicals Information Since 1932***

*Special Bibliographic Notes related to special journal issues (separates) and indexing/abstracting:*

- indexing/abstracting services in this list will also cover material in any "separate" that is co-published simultaneously with Haworth's special thematic journal issue or DocuSerial. Indexing/abstracting usually covers material at the article/chapter level.
- monographic co-editions are intended for either non-subscribers or libraries which intend to purchase a second copy for their circulating collections.
- monographic co-editions are reported to all jobbers/wholesalers/approval plans. The source journal is listed as the "series" to assist the prevention of duplicate purchasing in the same manner utilized for books-in-series.
- to facilitate user/access services all indexing/abstracting services are encouraged to utilize the co-indexing entry note indicated at the bottom of the first page of each article/chapter/contribution.
- this is intended to assist a library user of any reference tool (whether print, electronic, online, or CD-ROM) to locate the monographic version if the library has purchased this version but not a subscription to the source journal.
- individual articles/chapters in any Haworth publication are also available through the Haworth Document Delivery Service (HDDS).

As part of Haworth's continuing committment to better serve our library patrons, we are proud to be working with the following electronic services:

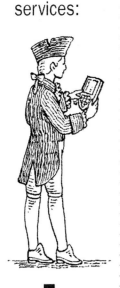

 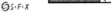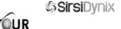

# Preventive Health Measures
# for Lesbian
# and Bisexual Women

## CONTENTS

# ABOUT THE EDITORS

**Shelly Kerr, PhD,** is the Assistant Director and Training Director and a licensed psychologist at the University of Oregon Counseling and Testing Center. Dr. Kerr earned her doctorate in Counseling Psychology from Washington State University. Shelly Kerr and Robin Mathy previously co-edited *Lesbian and Bisexual Women's Mental Health* (Haworth, 2005). Dr. Kerr was the author of several chapters included in that book on topics including bias in assessment and diagnosis of lesbian clients, depression and anxiety in lesbians, and mental health implications of same-sex marriage. Dr. Kerr's professional interests include LGBT issues, training and supervision, and multicultural issues (including white privilege).

**Robin Mathy, MA, MSc, MSW,** is a doctoral candidate in Evidence-Based Health Care at the University of Oxford. She is the author/editor of two previous books and over 50 peer-reviewed journal articles and book chapters. Her first work (co-authored with Frederick L. Whitam) *Male Homosexuality in Four Societies: Brazil, Guatemala, the Philippines, and the United States* (Praeger, 1986), has been continuously in print since its first publication, and is now included in the *New York Times Review of Books* as one of the best books in print in Anthropology. Robin Mathy and Shelly Kerr previously co-edited *Lesbian and Bisexual Women's Mental Health* (Haworth, 2005), and they are planning to co-edit a volume that addresses rural mental health and sexual minority issues. Robin's book *Gender Nonconformity & the Development of Homosexuality* will be published by Haworth next year. Robin earned an MSW in Clinical Research & Practice in Substance Abuse and Mental Health from the University of Minnesota, Twin Cities, where she also completed certificates in Child Abuse Prevention Studies and Drug & Alcohol Counseling. She also has earned an MSc in Evidence-Based Health Care from the University of Oxford, an MSt in International Relations from the University of Cambridge, an MA in Sociology from Indiana University-Bloomington, and she is completing an MEd in Family Education at the University of Minnesota, Twin Cities. She is on the Editorial Board of *Journal of Gay & Lesbian Psychotherapy* and a member of the International Academy of Sex Research.

# Preface

This is the second thematic volume we have edited together. While editing our earlier work, *Lesbian and Bisexual Women's Mental Health* (Haworth, 2005), we recognized the need to compile an edited volume about lesbian and bisexual women's physical health. As with our earlier work, *Preventive Health Measures for Lesbian and Bisexual Women* emphasizes evidence-based, empirical research that expands our understanding of health and medical issues that sexual minority women confront in everyday life. We chose *Preventive Health Measures* for its title because it signifies the subject of the work as well as its importance for the population about which contributors have conducted research and written. The Office on Women's Health, a component of the U.S. Department of Health and Human Services, reported that, "Lesbians face unique challenges within the health care system that can cause poor mental and physical health" (2006, p. 1). Several factors can become barriers to lesbian health care. First, lesbians and their health care providers may perceive a decreased risk of acquiring sexually transmitted infections and certain cancers (e.g., cervical cancer). Second, they may fear rejection, humiliation, discrimination, and oppression if they disclose their sexual orientation. Third, although cultural competence has become increasingly important to medical and health care practitioners and educators, providers must continuously strive to increase their knowledge, skills, and abilities regarding diverse populations, including lesbian and bisexual women. Lack of understanding can create perceptions of insensitivity and ignorance that become substantial barriers to acquiring health care long after a specific, adverse provider-patient interaction has ended. Finally, most states in the U.S., and indeed most

[Haworth co-indexing entry note]: "Preface." Kerr, Shelly, and Robin Mathy. Co-published simultaneously in *Women & Health* (The Haworth Medical Press, an imprint of The Haworth Press, Inc.) Vol. 44, No. 2, 2006, pp. xxiii-xxx; and: *Preventive Health Measures for Lesbian and Bisexual Women* (ed: Shelly Kerr, and Robin Mathy) The Haworth Medical Press, an imprint of The Haworth Press, Inc., 2006, pp. xix-xxvi. Single or multiple copies of this article are available for a fee from The Haworth Document Delivery Service [1-800-HAWORTH, 9:00 a.m. - 5:00 p.m. (EST). E-mail address: docdelivery@haworthpress.com].

countries in the world, do not afford lesbians the right to benefit from a partner's health insurance coverage. Recently, South Africa became the fifth country in the world to permit same-sex marriage. Yet the United States, which ironically was a worldwide leader in the fight against the South Africa's defunct policy of *Apartheid*, has continued to create barriers to same-sex marriage that would extend to a lesbian's partner the insurance coverage needed to benefit from preventive health care as well as medical treatment for disease. Consequently, lesbians frequently avoid preventive health care and procrastinate when medical care is needed (Office of Women's Health, p. 1).

The articles contributed in this work make it clear that the health of lesbian and bisexual women is important for health care providers and public health professionals. In her address to the Institute of Medicine's National Academy of Sciences Committee on Lesbian Health Research (1997) on behalf of the American Psychological Association, Charlotte Patterson, PhD noted a lack of information about lesbian and bisexual women's health. She attributed this problem, in part, to the paucity of health research focused on lesbian and bisexual women. Dr. Patterson made several recommendations to the Committee including addressing psychosocial and behavioral factors that have been neglected in health research and modifying research policies of the National Institute of Health and Center for Disease Control to include research on lesbian and bisexual women. Two years later, the Institute of Medicine (IOM) noted that the health issues of lesbian and bisexual women have been neglected for more than two decades (National Academy Press, 1999). In its work *Lesbian Health: Current Assessment and Directions for the Future*, IOM (1999) argued that lesbian health risks are associated with ongoing prejudice, discrimination, and the stigmatization of homosexuality in society at large. We addressed the mental health sequelae of prejudice, discrimination, and stigmatization in *Lesbian and Bisexual Women's Mental Health*. Even a cursory search in Medline or PsycInfo can identify a plethora of articles associated with these topics. However, evidence that societal-level discrimination, prejudice, and stigmatization can affect lesbian and bisexual women's physical health is more difficult to acquire. An effort to encourage lesbians to obtain pap tests (to obtain early detection of malignant cervical cells) was affected when radio advertisements in a "lesbian health matters" public health campaign led to listener complaints about hearing the word "lesbian" (Phillips-Angeles et al., 2004). Lesbian and bisexual women as well as gay and bisexual men and transgender adults reported that they perceived discrimination from administration and care staff in retirement care facilities (Johnson, Jackson, Arentte, & Koffman, 2005). The IOM also hypothesized that lesbian health may be affected by barriers to appropriate care, including "(1) structural barriers (e.g., availability of services, organizational configuration of health care providers); (2) financial barriers (e.g., insurance coverage); and (3) personal and cultural barriers (e.g., attitudes of patients and providers) (IOM, 1993)" (p. 37). Discrimination against lesbian, gay, and bisexual patients by physicians is well known, as is discrimination against lesbian, gay, or bisexual physicians by other health care professionals (Druzin, Shier, Yacowar, & Rossignol, 1998). Druzin et al. randomly sampled 500 individuals in a large urban city in Canada and obtained a sample of 346 participants, 41 of whom (11.8%) indicated they would refuse to see a gay, lesbian, or bisexual physician. They found no statistically significant difference in whether the physician was lesbian or gay. The websites of the Gay & Lesbian Medical Association, National Center for Lesbian Rights, and other national gay and lesbian rights organizations have documented a number of cases in which lesbians have been discriminated against by medical professionals.

This book is, in part, a response to the calls for more empirical, evidence-based research to address health care issues confronted by lesbian and bisexual women. Although we had hoped to acquire enough articles to produce a thematic double issue of *Women & Health* (and *Preventive Health Measures for Lesbian & Bisexual Women*), this proved to be a daunting task at this time, particularly with regard to the inclusion of lesbian and bisexual women of color. Thus, although this book represents a move forward in compiling a work that addresses lesbian and bisexual women's health, it focuses on preventive health. Greater efforts are needed to address the intersection of ethnicity and female sexual minority health. This is especially important because ethnically diverse women carry the oppression and disadvantage endemic to three minority groups: Women, lesbian, and ethnic diversity. Theoretically, to the extent that discrimination, oppression, and stigmatization affect health, we would expect sexual minority women to have greater risks than heterosexual women, and ethnically diverse lesbians to have greater risks than other sexual minority women. Conversely, one might reason that the discrimination, oppression, and stigma of growing up with a minority ethnic identity might mediate the adverse sequelae of developing a sexual minority identity. This is an important avenue of further research, and one the editors will explore as we continue to promote empirical, evidence-based research in our communities of lesbian and bisexual women.

Most of the health and medical research on lesbian and bisexual women has focused on samples of self-identified individuals. Little is known about the health differences between women who have sex with women (WSW) vis-à-vis those who identify as lesbian or bisexual. Is this important? Perhaps. As yet, we simply do not know. However, the phenomena of heterosexually identified women having sex with women has been prevalent enough (in recent years, at least) to warrant the publication of *Straight Girl's Guide to Sleeping with Chicks* (Sincero, 2005), which as of this writing ranks #4,314 in top sellers on Amazon.com. Thus, we would argue that research addressing "lesbian" and "bisexual" women's health issues must move toward inclusion of female same-sex behavior as well as studies of the relationships between bisexual or lesbian identity formation, health care utilization, and psychosocial, social structural, and cultural barriers to acquiring reliable, affordable health care.

Wells, Bimbi, Tider, Van Ora, and Parsons (Preventive Health Behaviors Among Lesbian and Bisexually Identified Women) contributed an article that emphasizes the importance of considering the potentially confounding effects of collapsing groups of lesbian vis-à-vis bisexual-identified women into a homogeneous whole. They also emphasized the potentially confounding effects of collapsing into a single group all women who have sex with women, some of whom do not identify as lesbian or bisexual. Because some health risk behaviors may be associated with the process of acquiring a bisexual or lesbian identity (see, for example, Gruskin et al., in this volume) rather than same-sex behavior among females per se, this is an important point. Conversely, risks of acquiring HIV may be endemic to same-sex behavior independent of identity, underscoring the need to give a priori methodological thought to designing a study in such a way that one's sample is drawn from the appropriate population of interest. The piece by Wells et al. complements quite nicely the contribution by Bowen et al. (this volume). From an evidence-based health care perspective, one must take care to account for variations in sampling methods as well as operational definitions for the population of interest. For example, however methodologically robust one may regard a random sample inclusive of women who have sex with women, the results cannot be generalized to self-identified lesbian and bisexual women. Indeed, Wells et al. make an excellent point in emphasizing the need to "carefully examine within group differences (lesbian vs. bisexual) to determine the exact nature of risk involved for women, and how sexual identity and behavior may factor in that risk."

Grindel, McGehee, Patsdaughter, and Roberts (Cancer Prevention and Screening Behaviors in Lesbians) contributed a valuable article about lesbian's compliance with the American Cancer Society's guidelines for cancer prevention and screening. Using a 102-item self-report instrument, they obtained a relatively large sample ($N = 1,139$) from 44 states in the U.S. Their data were gathered as part of the Boston Lesbian Health Project II, a replication of the first Boston Lesbian Health Project performed in 1987. This replication is important, in part, because it demonstrates persistence and continuity despite limited funding and public interest. Although the authors found that lesbians in the sample met most ACS guidelines, they noted that areas for behavioral improvement exist with regard to "nutrition, weight management, exercise, safer sex practices, sunscreen use and self-breast examination."

Boehmer and Case (Sexual Minority Women's Interactions with Breast Cancer Providers) also contributed to the lesbian health literature by identifying dimensions associated with sexual minority women's satisfaction with health care providers. Using a qualitative, grounded theory method, they interviewed 39 sexual minority women with breast cancer. They found that certain interpersonal behaviors as well as medical expertise and decision-making were associated with patient satisfaction. The authors' paper is rich with verbatim transcripts that elucidate quite elegantly some of the factors associated with sexual minority women's satisfaction with cancer care providers. This qualitative study complements the other papers included in this volume by demonstrating that empirical, evidence-based literature can include richly detailed, hermeneutic research that enhances our comprehension of the first-order meaning (to cancer survivors) of high-quality provider-patient care.

Sinding, Grassau, and Barnoff (Community Support, Community Values: The Experiences of Lesbians Diagnosed with Cancer) complements the work by Boehmer and Case. The authors provided another qualitative, empirical, evidence-based paper that enhances our understanding of the complex meanings of shared lesbian identity and participation in lesbian communities. They noted that shared lesbian identity is important but not always sufficient for obtaining social support; and, at times, it can be perceived as isolating and disquieting for various reasons, not the least of which is a generalized fear of cancer and perhaps exposure to another female whose "female" organs have been afflicted with cancer. This research can be helpful to public health professionals as well as social workers and clinicians working with lesbians diagnosed with or recovering from cancer. Given the importance of social support for illness prevention and health promotion, Sinding et al.'s work suggests that reliance upon lesbian networks for social support may be insufficient and possibly problematic. This has implications for further research in several disciplines, including Social Work and Community Psychology. To the extent that one's lesbian identity is salient, it would be reasonable to expect that she will seek support from other lesbians. However, it would be interesting (and perhaps important) to determine whether the salience of one's identity as a lesbian varies when social support is inadequate or problematic, particularly when confronting major life stressors and health issues.

Arena et al. (Psychosocial Responses to Treatment for Breast Cancer Among Lesbian and Heterosexual Women) compared 39 self-identified lesbians with a matched group of 39 heterosexual women, all of whom recently had been treated for breast cancer. Although the convenience sample is very small (and hence risks type II errors due to lack of statistical power), it provides additional insights into dynamics of social support from friends and family members as well as similarities and differences in coping styles among lesbians and heterosexual women treated for breast cancer. Friends and family members are important sources of social support, in addition to lesbian community for lesbian-identified women. However, social stigma and familial rejection associated with lesbian identity may compromise a key source of social support generally available to heterosexual women. Arena et al. suggest that lesbian women, relative to heterosexual peers, compensate for somewhat truncated social support from family members by increasing the social support received from friends. Given the results of Sinding et al.'s research, it would be important to ascertain whether the effect of social support from friends in general differs from receipt of social support from members of the lesbian community. It has been a longstanding methodological error to assume that lesbian identity is salient, and women for whom an identity as lesbian is less salient than other identities (e.g., mother, sister, friend, manager, nurse) may find it easier to compensate for deficient or problematic social support from lesbian community members by increasing social support received from heterosexual friends who have similar interests.

Gruskin, Byrne, Kools, and Altschuler (Consequences of Frequenting the Lesbian Bar) addressed the health risks associated with frequenting lesbian bars. Using a qualitative methodology, the authors recruited a sample of 35 self-identified lesbians, primarily from the San Francisco Bay area. Interestingly, the authors noted that connections to the lesbian community were fostered by attending bars, and this was an important part of lesbian identity development. In addition to being an important source of social support, lesbians in the study identified bars as a place to find sexual and intimate partners. Not unexpectedly, the authors discovered important health tradeoffs. For example, although frequenting lesbian bars increased social support, it could be associated with increased drug use. Conversely, binge drinking was offset by its community setting. In these contexts, the authors suggest the use of "harm reduction" strategies and redefining the lesbian bar to include the development of alternative social spaces in which to meet and socialize. As the research by Bowen, Bradford, and Powers (this volume) suggests, however, the location of a study and sampling design can (and often does) affect a study's findings. Several of the samples reported in *Lesbian and Bisexual Women's Mental Health* were obtained in a community-owned coffee house in Minneapolis, Minnesota, where many of the same functions of lesbian bars are fulfilled in a safe and sober venue. Nonetheless, this does not ameliorate the risks and benefits associated with frequenting lesbian bars in San Francisco, which has a long and culturally rich tradition in gay, lesbian, bisexual, and transgender communities.

In addition to theorizing that health-related behaviors may vary by lesbian identity salience, it is important to reflect upon methodological differences in study designs. Bowen, Bradford, and Powers (Comparing Sexual Minority Status Across Sampling Methods and Populations) empirically tested the hypothesis that variations in sampling methods may explain differences in health behavior rates among sexual minority women. They compared (a) a volunteer sample of women, (b) a volunteer sample of sexual minority women, (c) a population based telephone survey of women, and (d) an area probability sample of women. Relying upon their empirical, evidence-based data, the authors discuss the pros and cons of various sampling methods, with particular attention to reliability, ease of use, costs, and generalizability. Most importantly, their data substantiated the hypothesis that health risk behaviors among sexual minority women varied with sampling method. "This indicated that we need to use probability samples to base our estimates of health behavior performance. These types of estimates drive the national understanding of health disparities and are therefore important indicators of the health of a population." Nonetheless, the authors argue that convenience sampling is a viable alternative for some issues, such as obtaining a sample of sexual minority women willing to be assigned to various conditions of a randomized controlled trial or intervention. Matched control groups (see Arena et al., this volume) are another viable method for obtaining valid and reliable data. Of course, all research has limitations, and only careful appraisal of the relative contribution of each study to the composite whole of a corpus of research can enhance our ability to describe, explain, predict, and ultimately control health risks. As long as homosexuality is stigmatized, our ability to sample from (and generalize to) a population of lesbians, bisexual women, or both will be imperfect and imprecise.

In sum, this volume includes a combination of qualitative and quantitative articles, all of which are empirical and evidence-based. It is a small step toward advancing the goal of increasing the knowledge base regarding sexual minority women. Perhaps reflecting the major health concerns of sexual minority women, health care researchers, and/or funding agencies, many of the articles included here address cancer and preventive medicine. All of the articles underscore the meaning imbedded in the volume's title: *Preventive Health Measures for Lesbian and Bisexual Women*. It is our fervent hope that this volume will stimulate further empirical, evidence-based research regarding women who have sex with women as well as lesbian and bisexual-identified women across the lifecourse.

*Shelly Kerr, PhD*
*Robin Mathey, MA, MSc, MSW*

## REFERENCES

Committee on Lesbian Health Research Priorities, Institute of Medicine, National Academy of Sciences (1997). Testimony of Dr. Charlotte C. Patterson on Lesbian Health Research on behalf of the American Psychological Association. Retrieved June 26, 2006, from http://www.apa.org/pi/lgbc/publications/hltrsch.html.

Druzin, P., Shrier, I., Yacowar, M., & Rossignol, M. (1998). Discrimination against gay, lesbian and bisexual family physicians by patients. *Canadian Medical Association Journal, 158*(5), 593-597.

Institute of Medicine (1999). *Lesbian health: Current assessment and directions for the future.* Washington, D.C.: National Academy Press.

Johnson, M. J., Jackson, N. C., Arnette, J. K., & Koffman, S. D. (2005). Gay and lesbian perceptions of discrimination in retirement care facilities. *Journal of Homosexuality, 49*(2), 83-102.

Office on Women's Health, U.S. Department of Health & Human Services (2006). Lesbian Health. Retrieved November 30, 2006, from http://www.4woman.gov/faq/Lesbian.htm.

Phillips-Angeles, E., Wolfe, P., Myers, R., Dawson, P., Marrazzo, J., Soltner, S., & Dzieweczynski, M. (2004). Lesbian health matters: A pap test education campaign nearly thwarted by discrimination. *Health Promotion Practice, 5*(3), 314-325.

# Preventive Health Behaviors Among Lesbian and Bisexually Identified Women

Brooke E. Wells, MA
David S. Bimbi, PhD candidate
Diane Tider, MPH
Jason Van Ora, MA
Jeffrey T. Parsons, PhD

Brooke E. Wells and David S. Bimbi are affiliated with the Graduate Center of the City University of New York and the Center for HIV/AIDS Educational Studies and Training.

Diane Tider is affiliated with the Center for HIV/AIDS Educational Studies and Training.

Jason Van Ora is affiliated with the Graduate Center of the City University of New York.

Jeffrey T. Parsons is affiliated with Hunter College and the Graduate Center of the City University of New York and the Center for HIV/AIDS Educational Studies and Training.

Address correspondence to: Jeffrey T. Parsons, Professor, Hunter College of the City University of New York, Department of Psychology, 695 Park Avenue, New York, NY 10021 (E-mail: jeffrey.parsons@hunter.cuny.edu).

The authors acknowledge the contributions of other members of the Sex and Love Project team–Juline A. Koken, Joseph C. Punzalan, Jose Nanin, Joseph Severino, and Elana Rosof.

The Sex and Love Project was supported by the Hunter College Center for HIV/ AIDS Educational Studies and Training (CHEST), under the direction of Dr. Parsons.

[Haworth co-indexing entry note]: "Preventive Health Behaviors Among Lesbian and Bisexually Identified Women." Wells, Brooke E. et al. Co-published simultaneously in *Women & Health* (The Haworth Medical Press, an imprint of The Haworth Press, Inc.) Vol. 44, No. 2, 2006, pp. 1-13; and: *Preventive Health Measures for Lesbian and Bisexual Women* (ed: Shelly Kerr, and Robin Mathy) The Haworth Medical Press, an imprint of The Haworth Press, Inc., 2006, pp. 1-13. Single or multiple copies of this article are available for a fee from The Haworth Document Delivery Service [1-800-HAWORTH, 9:00 a.m. - 5:00 p.m. (EST). E-mail address: docdelivery@haworthpress.com].

**SUMMARY.** The current research aimed to better understand the preventive health behaviors of lesbian and bisexually identified women. We recruited lesbian and bisexual women at a large-scale Gay, Lesbian, and Bisexual (GLB) event in New York City. An ethnically diverse sample of 102 lesbian and 23 bisexually identified women who had sex with women from the New York City metropolitan area completed a quantitative survey. Lesbians, compared to bisexual women, were significantly older and significantly more likely to report being in partnered relationships. Lesbians were also more likely than bisexual women to report having performed recent breast self-examinations. Because of previously inconsistent findings and methodologies, further research is needed to determine the specific effects of lesbian or bisexual identity on preventive health behaviors. doi:10.1300/J013v44n02_01 *[Article copies available for a fee from The Haworth Document Delivery Service: 1-800-HAWORTH. E-mail address: <docdelivery@haworthpress.com> Website: <http://www. HaworthPress.com> © 2006 by The Haworth Press, Inc. All rights reserved.]*

**KEYWORDS.** Lesbian, bisexual, health behavior

Recent research has demonstrated the breadth of health epidemics, such as cardiovascular disease, breast cancer, and cervical cancer (National Center for Health Statistics, 2004). Studies have also shown that lesbians are at increased risk for breast and cervical cancers and at increased risk of mortality from these diseases (Gay and Lesbian Medical Association, 2001). Many think this may be a function of later detection of diseases (earlier detection generally predicts better prognosis), which results from lower rates of preventive health behaviors, such as Papanicolaou test screening (pap smear), breast self-exams, mammograms (Gay and Lesbian Medical Association, 2001). For example, recent research found that lesbian women are less likely to undergo annual pap smears and mammograms (Cochran et al., 2001; Diamant, Wold, Spritzer, & Gelberg, 2000), and breast self-exams (Rankow & Tessaro, 1998). However, other research shows no differences between lesbians and heterosexual women in undergoing preventive health care behaviors, such as routine annual mammograms (Aaron, Markovic, Danielson, Honnold, Janosky, & Schmidt, 2001; Koh, 2000) and cholesterol screening (Koh, 2000). These disparate results are difficult to reconcile, perhaps because of the differential measurement techniques and conceptualizations of sexual orientation.

Specifically, behavioral definitions of sexual orientation are often confounded with measurements that target identification (Diaz, Vlahov, Greenberg, Cuevas, & Garfein, 2001). On one end of the spectrum, sexual orientation is measured as a self-reported identity, and behavior is assumed to follow the reported sexual identity (e.g., lesbians have sex with women, heterosexual women have sex with men). In these studies, lesbians are often compared to heterosexual women, sometimes excluding bisexual women (e.g., Aaron et al., 2001), and other times collapsing lesbians and bisexuals into one group (i.e., Mays, Yancey, Cochran, Weber, & Fielding, 2002). On the other end of the spectrum, sexual orientation has been measured behaviorally, with all women who report sex with women being combined into one group (often called women who have sex with women or WSW), regardless of variance in sexual identity within that group (i.e., Marrazzo, Koutsky, Kiviat, Kuypers, & Stine, 2001; Fethers, Marks, Mindel, & Estcourt, 2000). While these studies seem to recognize the importance of not assuming sexual behaviors from a sexual identity category, they have gone to the opposite extreme of imposing sexual labels onto women based on their behaviors. In short, the literature often confounds behavioral and identity measures of sexual orientation.

While this makes comparison and literature review more difficult, evidence suggests within group variance that may be missed by combining WSW or lesbian/bisexual into one category. For example, Koh (2000) found differences in preventive health behaviors between bisexual and heterosexual women, with bisexual women being less likely to perform regular cholesterol and mammogram screenings, but did not find differences between lesbian and heterosexual women. On the other hand, Diamant et al. (2000) found that lesbians, but not bisexual women, were less likely than heterosexual women to have received annual pap smears and clinical breast examinations. These disparate findings make it even more important to carefully examine within group differences (lesbian vs. bisexual) to determine the exact nature of risk involved for women, and how sexual identity and behavior may factor into that risk. In addition to the empirical evidence against a one-dimensional measurement of sexual orientation, Young and Meyer (2005) point out that ignoring self-reported identity in favor of behavioral measurements undermines the community, networks, and relationships involved in a lesbian, gay, or bisexual (LGB) identity, consequently reducing a valid identity to a function of sexual behavior. Young and Meyer (2005) recommend that these behavioral measurements coincide with identity measures (rather than replace them) to provide a more accurate and nuanced picture.

The examination of sexual identity may be particularly important when examining health behaviors because identity may influence a variety of behaviors. Specifically, holding a lesbian identity may predict certain health behaviors through community involvement and support and/or through factors related to healthcare experiences. First, women who hold a lesbian identity may feel more involved with the lesbian community (as opposed to bisexual women, who are often stigmatized within both the lesbian community and the heterosexual community; Mulick & Wright, 2002). Consequently, these women may be exposed to health messages targeted to the lesbian community (i.e., The Lesbian Community Cancer Project–http://www.lccp.org/health/bse.html and efforts at state and local health departments–http://www.metrokc.gov/health/glbt/bcancer.htm) and might also experience social support within the lesbian community that may encourage preventive health behaviors. Secondly, in health care settings, women holding a lesbian identity may find it more relevant to disclose their sexual identity to their health care providers (HCPs) because the traditional gynecological examination so often responds to and focuses on heterosexual behavior. Bisexual women, assuming they are sexually active with both men and women, may find many of the assumptions about sexual behaviors to be more appropriate, thereby negating their need to clearly state their sexual identity and behavior. Women who disclose their sexual orientation are more likely to discuss a variety of health issues with their HCP, and consequently engage in more preventive health behaviors than their non-disclosing peers (White, 1998). Through both of these mechanisms, identity may prove to influence preventive health behaviors, such that lesbians might be more likely to engage in a variety of preventive health behaviors.

Recognizing the methodological limitations within those studies confounding behavior and identity and the importance of identity to health behaviors, we sought to expand on the notion that WSW is a heterogeneous population through an identification of potential demographic and preventive health behavior differences and similarities between lesbian-identified and bisexually-identified women who have sex with women. Moreover, we sought to understand whether lesbian-identified women who have sex with women would, in fact, report a higher rate of preventive health behaviors than bisexually identified women who have sex with women, thus demonstrating the influence of identity on behavior.

## METHOD

### Participants and Procedure

A cross-sectional, brief, street-intercept survey method (Miller, Wilder, Stillman, & Becker, 1997) was used to survey women at two large events targeting the gay, lesbian, bisexual and transgendered (GLBT) community in New York City in the Fall of 2002. This approach to collecting data has been used in numerous studies, including those focused on members of the GLBT community, and has been shown to provide data that is comparable to that obtained from other more methodologically rigorous approaches (Halkitis & Parsons, 2002; Koken, Parsons, Bimbi, & Severino, 2005) in which comparable rates of self-reported health behaviors have been found between samples derived from intercept surveys and those derived from random digit dialing.

At each two-day long event, the research team hosted a booth, and each woman who passed the booth was actively approached. Potential participants were provided with information about the project and offered the opportunity to participate. Participants were eligible if they verbally reported ever having sex with another woman. As an incentive, those who consented and completed the survey were provided with a voucher for free admission to a movie. To help ensure privacy, participants were given the survey on a clipboard so that they could step away from others while completing the questionnaire. The survey took approximately 10-15 minutes to complete and was completely confidential. Prior to completing the survey, participants were also given an assent form explaining the research and their rights as a research participant (a methodology approved by the last author's Institutional Review Board). Upon completion, participants deposited their own survey into a secure box at the booth. Data were later entered into an SPSS database and double-entered for accuracy. Any inconsistencies were reconciled by checking the completed survey.

### Measures

*Sociodemographics.* The survey included measures of several demographics, including: age (measured continuously), zip code, sexual identity (gay/lesbian, bisexual, or heterosexual/straight), HIV status (Positive, Negative, or Unknown), relationship status (Single or Partnered), and ethnicity (African American/African Descent, Asian/Pacific Islander, European/White, Hispanic/Latino, Middle Eastern/Arab, or Native American).

*Sexual Orientation.* Sexual identity was measured with a single self-report item asking women to check heterosexual, bisexual, or lesbian. For this particular survey, potential participants were only given the survey if they verbally disclosed past same-sex sexual behavior. Through these means, we were able to examine within WSW group differences (lesbian vs. bisexually-identified women).

*Preventive Health Behaviors.* Participants also reported their lifetime and recent (in the last year) experiences around having had a mammogram/clinical breast exam, breast self-exam, cholesterol screening, or pap smear (all dichotomously measured–yes/no).

## Data Analysis

All statistical analyses were conducted using SPSS Software version 12. First, we assessed demographic differences (race/ethnicity, sexual identity and relationship status) through ANOVAs for continuous variables and chi-square analyses for categorical variables. Those health behavior outcomes that differed significantly ($p < 0.05$) by sexual identity, were included in multiple logistic regression models to determine whether sexual identity was associated with preventive health behavior, after controlling for age and any other confounding variables. In the multiple logistic regression modelling, age went in the first step and sexual identity in the second step with the dichotomously coded preventive health behavior as the dependent variable using forward step conditional entry. Chi-square and Nagelkerke $R^2$ will be used to determine goodness of fit for the model and Wald criterion for individual variables. In this way, we could ascertain the independent influence of sexual identity after removing the variance associated with age.

## RESULTS

A total of 125 lesbian and bisexually identified women reporting any sexual activity with women consented to participate in the study. The response rate was high, with 83.4% of individuals approached consenting to participate. The majority ($n = 102$, 81.6%) were lesbian-identified women, while the remaining women ($n = 23$, 18.4%) identified as bisexual. The sample was ethnically diverse, with more than half ($n = 66$; 52.8%) identifying themselves as women of color (Table 1). The

TABLE 1. Demographics of Sample

| | Full Sample $n = 125$ | Lesbian $n = 102$ | Bisexual $n = 23$ |
|---|---|---|---|
| Age | 32.60 | 33.58 | 28.26* |
| | $(SD = 10.18)$ | $(SD = 10.12)$ | $(SD = 9.49)$ |
| Ethnicity | | | |
| African American | 16.8% | 15.7% | 21.7% |
| Asian/Pacific Islander | 6.4% | 5.9% | 8.7% |
| Latina | 20.8% | 20.6% | 21.7% |
| White | 47.2% | 49.0% | 39.1% |
| Mixed Race | 8.8% | 8.8% | 8.7% |
| Relationship Status | | | |
| Single | 34 (27.2%) | 24 (23.8%) | 10 (43.5%) |
| Partnered | 87 (69.6%) | 77 (76.2%) | 10 (43.5%)* |
| Not specified | 4 (3.2%) | 1 (1.0%) | 3 (13.0%) |

* Indicates a significant difference between lesbian and bisexual women, $p < .05$.

mean age of the women was 32.63 years ($SD = 10.23$; range = 18 to 67 years). The majority of the sample also reported being partnered ($n = 87$, 69.6%) as well as being HIV negative ($n = 94$, 75.2%; Unknown HIV status, $n = 18$, 14.4%; 1 woman was HIV positive, and the rest refused to answer). Not including HIV, almost a fifth of the women ($n = 24$, 19.2%) reported ever having a sexually transmitted infection (STI).

Bisexual women were significantly younger than lesbians (28.26 vs. 33.58 years, $F(1,123) = 5.3, p = 0.023$). No significant differences were observed between lesbians and bisexuals with regard to racial or ethnic identification. However, lesbians were 3.2 times more likely to report being partnered ($p = 0.017$; 95% CI = 1.19, 8.62). Bisexual women were 2.87 times more likely to report ever having contracted a STI ($p = 0.036$; 95% CI = 1.04, 7.87)

In terms of preventive health behaviors, results indicated that lesbians were significantly more likely to report having performed a breast self-exam in the last year. Conversely, bisexual women were more likely to report having ever or recently had cholesterol screening. No other significant differences in health screening behaviors emerged (Table 2). Race, relationship status and STI history were unrelated to

TABLE 2. Differences Between Lesbian and Bisexual Preventive Health Experiences

| Health Behaviors | Occurrence | Lesbians | Bisexuals | OR | 95% CI |
|---|---|---|---|---|---|
| Mammogram/ Clinical Breast Exam | Ever | 63.7% (n = 65) | 65.2% (n = 15) | 1.07 | .413-2.76 |
| | Past year | 36.3% (n = 33) | 45.0% (n = 9) | 1.43 | .540-3.83 |
| Pap Smear | Ever | 85.3% (n = 87) | 82.6% (n = 19) | 1.22 | .364-4.1 |
| | Past year | 60.2% (n = 56) | 71.4% (n = 15) | 1.65 | .587-4.64 |
| Breast Self Exam | Ever | 82.4% (n = 84) | 65.2% (n = 15) | 2.49 | .917-6.76 |
| | Past year* | 72.2% (n = 65) | 40.0% (n = 8) | 3.90 | 1.42-10.60 |
| Cholesterol Screening | Ever* | 51.0% (n = 52) | 73.9% (n = 17) | 2.72 | .994-7.49 |
| | Past year* | 31.6% (n = 32) | 60.0% (n = 14) | 3.25 | 1.20-8.78 |

*$p < .05$

these preventive health behaviors. However, women who performed breast self-exams in the last year were significantly older (34.4 vs. 29.4 years, $F(1,108) = 5.95$, $p = 0.016$).

As bisexual women were significantly younger, and women who performed breast self exams in the last year were significantly older, multiple logistic regression was then conducted for this outcome behavior, entering age first and then sexual identity (Table 3). A test of the full model (with both age and sexual identity as independent variables) against a constant-only model was statistically reliable, $\chi^2 (2) = 11.43$, $p < 0.01$, indicating that the independent variables, as a set, reliably distinguished between those who had and had not performed breast self-exams in the last year. The variance in performing breast self-exams for which these variables accounted was moderate, with Nagelkerke's $R^2 = .137$, indicating that age and sexual identity accounted for 13.7% of the variance in recent breast self-examination practices. In the final model, according to the Wald criterion, both age ($z = 3.82$, $p = 0.051$) and sexual identity ($z = 5.14$, $p = 0.023$) were associated with performing a breast self-exam in the last year, although sexual identity was more strongly associated. With the impact of age modeled in the equation, odds ratios indicated that lesbian women were more than three times as likely as bisexual women to have performed a recent breast self-exam (OR = 3.30).

TABLE 3. Logistic Regression Predicting Recent Breast Self Exam

| Variable | b | S.E | Wald | p | OR | Nagelkerke $R^2$ |
|---|---|---|---|---|---|---|
| Step 1 | | | | | | |
|    Age | .053 | .023 | 5.46 | .019 | 1.06 | .076 |
| Step 2* | | | | | | |
|    Age | .046 | .023 | 3.82 | .051 | 1.05 | .137 |
|    Sexual Identity | 1.197 | .528 | 5.137 | .023 | 3.31 | |

*$\Delta R^2$, p < .05

## DISCUSSION

Overall, these results indicated relatively high rates of lifetime preventive health behaviors, with at least 50% of all women reporting ever having engaged in a variety of preventive health behaviors. However, compared to lifetime rates, women reported much lower rates of recent preventive health behaviors, possibly indicating that lesbian and bisexual women are not engaging in regular or routine preventive health behaviors. These rates compare unfavorably to recent national rates for women. For example, the Morbidity and Mortality Weekly Report (MMWR, 2003) indicated that in 2001, 90% of women reported ever having a Pap smear (compared with 82.6-85.3% of our sample) and that 87.1% reported having a Pap smear in the preceding 3 years (compared with our 60.2-71.4% in the preceding year from our sample). However, these rates varied by age and by race and ethnicity, with women of color and younger women being less likely to have received a Pap smear.

In the present study, five major differences between lesbian and bisexual women emerged. Demographically, compared to bisexuals, the lesbians in this sample were generally older, more likely to report being in a partnered relationship, and less likely to have ever contracted an STI. In terms of preventive health behaviors, compared to bisexual women, lesbian-identified women were more likely to have performed breast self-examinations, even after controlling for age. Conversely, bisexual women were more likely than lesbians to have undergone cholesterol screening, ever and recently. These disparate findings contradict (Rankow & Tessaro, 1998) and move beyond the available literature, illustrating the need for further research and a clear delineation of the effects of behavior and identity.

A number of explanations might adequately account for these results. First, lesbians may be more aware of the need for breast self-exams because of ongoing efforts to educate the lesbian community about the need for early detection (for example, the Mautner Project, *www. mautnerproject.org*, which provides outreach and information about breast cancer to the lesbian community). Because of their involvement in the lesbian community (attending events, reading lesbian centered magazines, socializing with other lesbians, etc.), these women may have been exposed to these educational messages. On the other hand, bisexuals may not be as involved in the community because they have traditionally been stigmatized within the lesbian community (Mulick & Wright, 2002). Consequently, they may not have been as exposed to these messages or received the social support from the lesbian community that might also encourage breast self-examination. Alternatively, the lesbian-bisexual difference may be a function of the relationship between identity and disclosure to a HCP. It may be that lesbians feel that their sexual identity is a more salient aspect of their identity in health care situations, which may lead them to disclose their sexual orientation to their HCP. Disclosure of sexual orientation to the HCP increases communication between the woman and her HCP, which also leads women to discuss preventive health behaviors and other lifestyle choices with her HCP and may also lead the HCP to intentionally promote preventive health behaviors (White, 1998). This latter explanation, though, may not account for the difference in cholesterol screening. This result may also be a factor of community exposure to messages about preventive health behaviors. While the lesbian community has been inundated with messages about breast cancer, other preventive health messages may have been neglected. Clearly, future research should more closely examine the complex relationship between sexual identity and preventive health behaviors and the underlying mechanisms that guide this relationship.

As with most studies, methodological limitations in the present study prevent clearer conclusions about the relationships postulated. Because we used a brief street-intercept survey methodology, we were reliant on self-report of health care behaviors, so that women may have provided more socially acceptable responses, which may have resulted in an overestimate of health behaviors. We may also have introduced self-selection bias, in that those who attended a GLBT event and consented to participate in the survey may have been demographically or otherwise distinct from those who did not attend or who refused. Additionally, this convenience sample included only a relatively small group of women who attended a large-scale GLB event, which prevents generalization to the broader population of lesbian and bisexual women. More importantly, this survey, because it was designed to be a very brief street-intercept survey, did not assess a variety of factors that may have played a role in the relationship between sexual identity and preventive health behaviors. For example, differences between lesbians and bisexuals in socioeconomic status may have influenced preventive health behaviors because of limited access to healthcare. Educational attainment may have also influenced the observed differences by determining the level of knowledge of the need for preventive health behaviors. Additionally, several factors (i.e. access to healthcare, past experiences, and lifestyle factors, such as smoking and physical activity) may be related to the level of disclosure to and comfort with HCPs, which could, in turn, influence a variety of preventive health behaviors. Finally, this study was limited because the measures used were original measures and have not been previously validated in an LGB sample.

Despite these limitations, this study provides evidence that it is essential to acknowledge differences in health behaviors related to women's sexual identities so that researchers and health practitioners can be aware of and identify the relationships among sexual behavior, sexual identity, and preventive health behaviors. Additionally, this research demonstrates that it is essential to consider other factors (i.e., age) that may be influencing these relationships. Future research is needed to determine the extent to which a lesbian identity might be influencing preventive health behaviors through various mechanisms, such as educational attainment, access to care, social support, community involvement, and relationship with HCPs. It is essential that behavioral health researchers continue to investigate the impact of sexual identity on health risk and health prevention behaviors, working toward the development of interventions that accurately target and support diverse groups of women.

## REFERENCES

Aaron, D.J., Markovic, N., Danielson, M.E., Honnold, J.A., Janosky, J.E., & Schmidt, N.J. (2001). Behavioral risk factors for disease and preventive health practices among lesbians. *American Journal of Public Health, 91*, 972-975.

Centers for Disease Control and Prevention. *Surveillance Summaries*, August 22, 2003. MMWR 2003: 52 (No. SS-8). Accessed online on February 21, 2006 at *www.cdc.gov/mmwr/PDF/ss/ss5208.pdf.*

Cochran, S.D., Mays, V.M., Bowen, D., Gage, S., Bybee, D. Roberts, S.J., Goldstein, R.S., et al. (2001). Cancer-related risk indicators and preventive screening behaviors among lesbians and bisexual women. *American Journal of Public Health, 91,* 591-597.

Diamant, A.L., Wold, C., Spritzer, K., & Gelberg, L. (2000). Health behaviors, health status, and access to and use of health care: A population-based study of lesbian, bisexual, and heterosexual women. *Archives of Family Medicine, 9,* 1043-1051.

Diaz, T., Vlahov, D., Greenberg, B., Cuevas, Y., & Garfein, R. (2001). Sexual orientation and HIV infection prevalence among young Latino injection drug users in Harlem. *Journal of Women's Health & Gender Based Medicine, 10,* 371-380.

Fethers, K., Marks, C., Mindel, A., & Estcourt, C.S. (2000). Sexually transmitted infections and risk behaviors in women who have sex with women. *Sexually Transmitted Infections, 76,* 345-349.

Gay and Lesbian Medical Association and LGBT Health Experts. *Healthy People 2010 Companion Document for Lesbian, Gay, Bisexual, and Transgender (LGBT) Health.* San Francisco, CA: Gay and Lesbian Medical Association, 2001. Accessed online on October 13, 2005 at *http://www.glma.org/policy/hp2010/PDF/HP2010CDLGBTHealth.pdf.*

Halkitis, P. N., & Parsons, J. T. (2002). Recreational drug use and HIV-risk sexual behavior among men frequenting gay social venues. *Journal of Gay & Lesbian Social Services, 14,* 19-38.

Kennedy, M.B., Scarlett, M.I., Duerr, A.C., & Chu, S.Y. (1995). Assessing HIV risk among women who have sex with women: Scientific and communication issues. *Journal of the American Women's Association, 50,* 103-107.

Koh, A.S. (2000). Use of preventive health behaviors by lesbian, bisexual, and heterosexual women: Questionnaire survey. *Western Journal of Medicine, 172,* 379-384.

Koken, J.A., Parsons, J.T., Bimbi, D.S., & Severino, J. (2005). Exploring commercial sex encounters in an urban community sample of gay and bisexual men: A Preliminary report. *Journal of Psychology and Human Sexuality, 17,* 197-213.

Kral, A.H., Lorvick, J., Bluthenthal, R.N., & Watters, J.K. (1997). HIV risk profile of drug-using women who have sex with women in 19 United States cities. *Journal of Acquired Immune Deficiency Syndromes & Human Retrovirology, 16,* 211-217.

Lesbian Community Cancer Project. Accessed online on October 13, 2005 at: *http://www.lccp.org/health/bse.html*

Marrazzo, J.M., Koutsky, L.A., Kiviat, N.B., Kuypers, J.M., & Stine, K. (2001). Papanicolaou test screening and prevalence of genital human papillomavirus among women who have sex with women. *American Journal of Public Health, 91,* 947-952.

Mays, V.M., Yancey, A.K., Cochran, S.D., Weber, M., & Fielding, J.E. (2002). Heterogeneity of health disparities among African American, Hispanic, and Asian American women: Unrecognized influences of sexual orientation. *American Journal of Public Health, 92,* 632-639.

Miller, K.W., Wilder, L.B., Stillman, F.A., & Becker, D.M. (1997). The feasibility of a street-intercept survey method in an African-American community. *American Journal of Public Health, 87,* 655-658.

Mulick, P.S. & Wright, L.W. (2002). Examining the existence of biphobia in the heterosexual and homosexual populations. *Journal of Bisexuality, 2,* 45-64.

National Center for Health Statistics. Health, United States, 2004 with Chartbook on Trends in the Health of Americans. Hyattsville, Maryland: 2004. Accessed online on October 13, 2005 at: *http://www.cdc.gov/nchs/data/hus/hus04.pdf.*

Rankow, E.J. & Tessaro, I (1998). Mammography and risk factors for breast cancer in lesbian and bisexual women. *American Journal of Health Behavior, 22,* 403-410.

Seattle & King County Public Health Department. Accessed online on October 13, 2005 at: *http://www.metrokc.gov/health/glbt/bcancer.htm*

White, J.C. (1998). Room for improvement: Communication between lesbians and their primary care providers. In *Gateways to Improving Lesbian Health and Health Care: Opening Doors.* Ed. by Ponticelli, C.M. Binghamton, NY: The Harrington Park Press/The Haworth Press, Inc.

Young, R.M. & Meyer, I.H. (2005). The trouble with "MSM" and "WSW": Erasure of the sexual-minority person in public health discourse. *American Journal of Public Health, 95,* 1144-1149.

doi:10.1300/J013v44n02_01

# Cancer Prevention and Screening Behaviors in Lesbians

Cecelia Gatson Grindel, PhD, RN, CMSRN, FAAN
Linda A. McGehee, PhD, RN
Carol A. Patsdaughter, PhD, RN
Susan J. Roberts, DNSc, RN, ANP

**SUMMARY.** The incidence of cancer diagnosis has increased in the United States highlighting the need for astute cancer prevention and screening behaviors. Previous literature has suggested that lesbians may not follow the American Cancer Society's (ACS) guidelines regarding prevention and screening for cancer due to disparity in access to care and increased use of alcohol and tobacco. The purpose of this study was to examine the cancer prevention and screening behaviors of lesbians using the ACS guidelines as the standards for comparison, and to determine factors that influence mammography screening.

A 102-item self-report survey was distributed to lesbians nationwide

---

Cecelia Gatson Grindel is Associate Director for Graduate Programs, Georgia State University, Atlanta, GA.

Linda A. McGehee is Assistant Professor, Georgia State University, Atlanta, GA.

Carol A. Patsdaughter is Visiting Professor, Florida International University, North Miami, FL.

Susan J. Roberts is Associate Professor, Northeastern University, Boston, MA.

Address correspondence to: Cecelia Gatson Grindel, PhD, RN, CMSRN, FAAN, Associate Director for Graduate Programs, Professor, Georgia State University, P.O. Box 4019, Atlanta, GA 30302-4019.

[Haworth co-indexing entry note]: "Cancer Prevention and Screening Behaviors in Lesbians." Grindel, Cecelia Gatson et al. Co-published simultaneously in *Women & Health* (The Haworth Medical Press, an imprint of The Haworth Press, Inc.) Vol. 44, No. 2, 2006, pp. 15-39; and: *Preventive Health Measures for Lesbian and Bisexual Women* (ed: Shelly Kerr, and Robin Mathy) The Haworth Medical Press, an imprint of The Haworth Press, Inc., 2006, pp. 15-39. Single or multiple copies of this article are available for a fee from The Haworth Document Delivery Service [1-800-HAWORTH, 9:00 a.m. - 5:00 p.m. (EST). E-mail address: docdelivery@haworthpress.com].

*15*

using various methods including snowballing sampling techniques. The sample included 1139 self-identified lesbians from 44 states.

In general, healthy lifestyle behaviors were followed. The majority of the women did not smoke, ate plenty of fruits and vegetables, ate protein sources low in fat and consumed alcohol at a moderate rate. However, safe sex practices were often not used by participants. Most women did have mammograms and Papanicolaou smears (PAP) as recommended; however, adherence to self-breast examination guidelines was not followed. Women who were older, had higher yearly incomes, did not smoke, performed regular self breast exams and had regular physical exams were most likely to have a mammogram.

Over half of the women met American Cancer Society guidelines for prevention and screening for breast and cervical cancer. However, strategies are needed to increase compliance with these guidelines in order to improve cancer health outcomes. doi:10.1300/J013v44n02_02 *[Article copies available for a fee from The Haworth Document Delivery Service: 1-800-HAWORTH. E-mail address: <docdelivery@haworthpress.com> Website: <http://www.HaworthPress.com> © 2006 by The Haworth Press, Inc. All rights reserved.]*

**KEYWORDS.** Cancer screening, health promotion, healthy lifestyles, lesbians

The incidence of cancer diagnosis has increased in the United States highlighting the need for astute cancer prevention and screening behaviors. Previous literature has suggested that lesbians may be at higher risk for cancer as they use alcohol and cigarettes more than heterosexual women (Roberts & Sorensen, 1999; Valanis, Bowen, Bassford, Whitlock, Charney, & Carter, 2000) and may not follow the American Cancer Society's Guidelines for Early Detection of Cancer (Smith, Cokkinides, Eyre, 2003) regarding screening for cervical cancer (Diamant, Schuster, & Lever, 2000; Rankow & Tessaro, 1998). The purpose of this study was to examine the cancer prevention and screening behaviors of lesbians in light of the American Cancer Society's guidelines related to cancer prevention and screening. Specifically, the aims of this project were to (1) describe cancer prevention behaviors (nutrition, exercise, tobacco use, alcohol consumption, safe sex practices, sunscreen use); (2) explore screening behaviors related to breast and gynecological health; and (3) examine factors that influence mammography screening in lesbians.

# BACKGROUND

*Smoking:* Reports of tobacco use in lesbians have shown varied results. Aaron, Markovic, Danielson, Honnold, Janosky, and Schmidt (2001) reported that lesbians in their sample were more likely to smoke (35.5%) than women in the general population (20.3%) who were surveyed for the 1998 Behavior Risk Factor Surveillance System (BRFSS). An extensive review of the literature by Hughes and Jacobson (2003) indicated that lesbians were more likely to smoke than heterosexual women. In several studies, smoking rates among lesbians has been reported between 11-28% (Burnett, Steakley, Slack, Roth, & Lerman, 1999; Diamant et al., 2000; Rankow and Tessaro, 1998; Roberts & Sorenson, 1999; Valanis et al., 2000; White and Dull, 1997). In contrast, a meta-analysis of seven studies from 1989-1995 indicated that lesbians appeared to be less likely to smoke in comparison to United States women in general (Cochran, Mays, Bowen, Gage, Bybee, Roberts, Goldstein, Robison, Rankow, & White, 2001). Roberts, Dibble, Scanlon, Paul, and Davids (1998) also documented that heterosexuals were more likely to report current tobacco use.

*Nutrition, Weight and Exercise:* Few lesbian health studies describe nutritional status. Valanis et al. (2000) reported lower intake of fruit and vegetables compared with heterosexual women. Roberts and Sorensen (1999) documented that 80% (n = 1306) of the participants "sometimes" or "regularly" ate breakfast and consumed high fiber diets. Related to nutrition, obesity has been cited as a common problem in lesbians (Aaron et al., 2001; Cochran et al., 2001, Roberts et al. 1998); however, lesbian and bisexual women as a whole were less likely to consider themselves as having a weight problem (Cochran et al., 2001). Physical activity is closely related to diet and weight. Roberts and Sorensen (1999) reported that lesbians exercised more than heterosexual women. According to Aaron et al. (2001), little difference in physical activity existed between lesbian and heterosexual women, however, a higher percentage of lesbians described engaging in vigorous activity. Valanis et al. (2000) reported that 30.3% of lifetime lesbians and 21.6% of adult lesbians in their study participated in four or more moderate to strenuous exercise activities per week, while 26.9% of the heterosexual respondents reported a similar exercising pattern.

*Alcohol Use:* Several researchers addressed alcohol use among lesbians. Most reports indicated that lesbians more often used alcohol (Bradford, Ryan, & Rothblum, 1994; Rankow & Tessaro, 1998; Roberts & Sorensen, 1999; Valanis et al., 2000). Roberts et al. (1998) found no significant differences between lesbian and heterosexual women in current or past alcohol use, history of blackouts, or alcohol problems. Other studies only reported on alcohol usage. In several studies the majority of the sample reported some use of alcohol (Aaron et al., 2001; Diamont et al., 2000; White & Dull, 1997). Some investigators reported that a small percent of lesbians (4-6% of their sample) could be classified as heavy drinkers (Aaron et al., 2001; Bradford et al., 1994; Roberts & Sorensen, 1999). In Cochran and associates' (2001) review of 7 research studies on cancer risks and screening behaviors among lesbians, 69.6% of the lesbians currently drank alcohol compared with 66.9% of U.S. women.

*Hormone Replacement Therapy:* The literature is scarce in reports about the use of hormone replacement (HRT) by lesbians. However, Valanis et al. (2000) documented that lesbian, bisexual, and heterosexual women had similar rates of using HRT (66%-71%). Two studies reported no statistically significant differences in HRT use between lesbians and heterosexual women (Dibble, Roberts, Robertson, & Paul, 2002; Roberts et al., 1998).

*Safe Sex Practices:* Little has been written on "safe sex" practices of lesbians. In a study of 78 lesbians, Fishman and Anderson (2003) reported that 53% of the lesbians indicated they were at low risk for contracting human immunodeficiency virus (HIV). These women reported knowledge of barrier methods to safe sex practices; however, 35%-40% had no knowledge of less common safe sex practices. Diamont et al. (2000) reported that 4993 lesbians (72%) reported lifetime histories of vaginal intercourse. Of these women, 4443 (89%) reported lifetime histories of vaginal intercourse without condom use. In Koh's study of 1,161 women (2000), lesbians ($n$ = 524; 45%) were more likely than heterosexual women ($n$ = 637; 55%) to practice safe sex (odds ratio 2.60, 95% confidence interval 1.23 to 5.49). Carroll, Goldstein, Lo, and Mayer (1997) provided more specific information about the use of protection among lesbians and bisexual women in Massachusetts. In female-to-male encounters, a lack of protection was reported by 34% of the women experiencing penile-vaginal penetration and 40.6% engaging in penile-anal penetration. Genital-genital contact occurred with male partners without protection in nearly 30% of the group. In sexual encounters with other women, protection was often not used when engaging in specific sexual behaviors: digital-vaginal (82.4%), oral-genital (78.6%), and genital-genital (70.1%). This report did not include information about perceived risk by respondents in light of their personal relationship with their sexual partners.

*Sunscreen Use:* No studies were found on the use of sunscreen by lesbians or women in general. However, other studies reported sunscreen use between 35% and 76% in their samples (Johnson & Lookingbill, 1984; Pruim, Wright, & Green, 1999; Robinson, Rigel, & Amonette, 1997). Individuals with higher income and education levels were likely to use sunscreen (Purdue, 2002).

## Breast Cancer Screening

*Mammography:* In general, research has suggested that lesbians have fairly high rates of following the recommended mammography screening guidelines with 58-84% of the lesbians reporting having a mammogram within one to two years (Burnett et al., 1999; Diamont et al., 2000; Lauver et al., 1999; Rankow and Tessaro, 1998; Roberts & Sorensen, 1999; Valanis et al., 2000). The rates for mammography screening participation were even higher (94%) for those at increased risk for breast cancer due to family history (Burnett et al., 1999).

In the Epidemiologic Study of Health Risk in Lesbians (ESTHER), Aaron et al. (2001) reported that, compared with the BRFSS sample, lesbians 40 years or older were more likely ever to have had a mammogram (93.3%; 95% CI = 91.3, 95.3) than their heterosexual counterparts, and lesbians 50 years or older were more likely to have had a mammogram within the past two years (88.1%; 95% CI = 84.2, 92.0). In their study on cancer risk factors, Cochran and colleagues (2001) noted that lesbians ages 40-49 were less likely to have a mammogram ($n$ = 2808, 73.1%) than estimated for all U.S. women (95% CI = 86.7%, 83.4, 89.9). Roberts et al. (1998) found no significant differences between lesbians ($n$ = 186, 43%) and heterosexual women ($n$ = 236, 40.3%) ever having had a mammogram.

In the studies above, mammography screening rates for lesbians ranged from 58% to 84%. Recent data on screening rates for women in general reported by the Centers for Disease Control and Prevention indicated that 70.3% of women 40 years and over had a mammogram in the past two years (National Center for Health Statistics, 2004). Recent studies indicate that mammogram screening rates are comparable and have increased for women in general and lesbians (Cochran et al., 2001; Diamont et al., 2000; Lauver et al., 1999; National Center for Health Statistics, 2004; Rankow & Tessaro, 1998; Roberts et al., 1998; Roberts & Sorensen, 1999).

Several studies reported profiles of lesbians who were most likely to have a mammogram. Rankow and Tessaro (1998) reported that women age 40 and older who were white (p = .0001), had health insurance (p = .04), and had higher incomes (p = .02) were more likely to have ever had a mammogram. In another study of 139 lesbians, multivariate logistic regression analysis indicated that only income level and degree of breast cancer worries were positively and significantly associated with mammography adherence (Burnett et al., 1999). Lairson, Chan, and Newmark (2005) reported on the profile of 3,415 women veterans who were most likely to use mammography screening. Education, income, insurance and perceived risk of breast cancer were positively related to the use of mammography, whereas age, smoking, travel and appointment waiting time were inversely related to likelihood of mammography screening. Mammography use in urban African American women (N = 576) has been documented at a rate of 75% (*n* = 432). Key factors associated with mammography screening in these women included health status, basic knowledge of breast cancer screening guidelines, more education, insurance coverage, having a usual source for medical care and having a PAP test within the past three years (Greene, Torio, & Klassen, 2005).

*Self Breast Exam (SBE):* Few studies reported on lesbians' use of SBE. Rankow and Tessaro (1998) reported that most women in their study (*n* = 493; 86.5%) practiced SBE but only 29% (*n* = 165) did so at least monthly, compared with 38% of respondents in a national sample (Vital and Health Statistics, 1993). Slightly higher rates were reported among lesbians in other studies (Burnett et al., 1999; Roberts & Sorensen, 1999). Rankow and Tessaro (1998) noted that women with higher education (p = < .0001) and incomes (.02) were more likely to say they conducted SBE.

*Clinical Breast Exam (CBE):* In a study of 139 lesbians, Burnett and colleagues (1999) reported that 88% (*n* = 123) of the women adhered to the ACS clinical breast exam guidelines. They also noted that if an individual reported age-specific adherence to mammography, a vast majority also reported adherence to CBE (84% and 93% respectively), while only 38% adhered to SBE.

### Cervical Cancer Screening

*Papanicolaou Testing:* Reports on screening patterns for cervical cancer have varied across studies. Several studies published during the 1980's reported a range of 48%-55% of the lesbian participants having an annual PAP smear (Bradford & Ryan, 1988; Johnson, Guenther, Laube, & Keetel, 1981; Johnson, Smith, & Guenther 1987). Sample sizes for these studies ranged from 117 to 1925 women. Studies in the 1990's reported annual PAP smear rates among lesbians at 38-68% (Diamont et al., 2000; Rankow and Tessaro, 1998; Roberts and Sorensen, 1999; Valanis et al., 2000; White and Dull, 1997). In their 1998 report, Rankow and Tessaro (1998) noted that 43.5% (*n* = 223) of their sample of lesbian and bisexual women had a PAP test within the last year, compared with 67% of all women in North Carolina. Their finding demonstrated that lesbians were less likely to have PAP smears than their heterosexual counterparts. More recently, the results of a cross-sectional study of 1010 self-identified lesbians indicated that there was little difference between the lesbians and the general population of women in the proportion reporting ever having a PAP test (Aaron et al., 2001). Cochran et al. (2001) compared national estimates for women with five independently conducted surveys of lesbians/bisexual women (N = 11, 876). These researchers estimated that approximately 85% (95%; CI = 83.2%, 86.2%) of lesbians had had a pelvic examination in the previous five years.

In the studies presented above, the percentage of lesbians reporting an annual PAP test varied across studies ranging from 38% to 68%. In most cases PAP screening was not reported by age groups. In comparison, a recent study from the Centers for Disease Control and Prevention indicated that 81.3% of women 18 years and older had a PAP smear within the past three years (National Center for Health Statistics, 2004).

Previous literature has suggested that lesbians may be at higher risk for cancer as they may not follow the American Cancer Society's guidelines for cancer prevention and early detection, including the guidelines for screening for breast and cervical cancers. The purpose of the present study was to examine the cancer prevention and screening behaviors of lesbians in light of the American Cancer Society's guidelines related to cancer prevention and screening.

## *METHODS*

This project, the Boston Lesbian Health Project II (BLHP II), was a replication of the 1987 Boston Lesbian Health Project I (BLHP I). Women who self-identified as lesbians and were eighteen years or older were included in the study. The 102-item self-report survey was distributed nationwide using various methods such as flyers at clinics, bookstores, etc., advertisements in newsletters to lesbian audiences, and snowballing sampling techniques.

*Instrument:* The survey consisted of questions about personal health, family health history, nutrition, exercise, cancer screening, safe sex, and risk for HIV. The original questionnaire was developed by the researchers from the BLHP I (Roberts & Sorensen, 1999). All items from the original questionnaire were included in the survey; questions related to nutrition and HIV risk were added. This article focuses on cancer screening and prevention behaviors.

*Analysis:* SPSS version 11.5 (SPSS, Inc., 2002) was used to analyze the data. Descriptive analyses (means, standard deviation, frequencies, and percentages) were used to describe sample characteristics and summarize questionnaire data. Forward stepwise multiple logistic regression was conducted to determine which independent variables (age, education, income, smoking, routine physical exams, and self breast exams) were associated with mammography screening for women 40 years of age and older. These six variables were selected because they were associated with mammography screening in the literature. All six variables were retained in the stepwise multiple logistic regression analysis based on significant bivariate correlations ($p < .05$) with the dependent variable (routine mammography screening). Three variables (education, income, and smoking) were eliminated because they were no longer statistically significant in the multivariate model. Regression results indicated the overall model that included age, routine physical exam and self breast exam was statistically reliable in distinguishing between women over 40 years old who had regular mammography screening and those who did not ($-2$ Log Likelihood = 425.682). Goodness-of-Fit statistic was tested by the Hosmer-Lemeshow Test; $\chi^2$ (8) = 7.57, p = .476. Nonsignificant $p$ values indicate that the model does fit the data (Munro, 2005). However, only 8.6% (Cox & Snell $R^2$) to 12.5% (Nagelkerte $R^2$) of the variance was accounted for in the multiple logistic regression model.

## RESULTS

*Sample:* The sample consisted of 1139 lesbians from 44 states. The state with the largest representation in the study was Massachusetts ($n = 276$; 24.8%), followed by California ($n = 85$; 7.6%), Georgia ($n = 62$; 5.6%), and Texas ($n = 52$; 4.7%). The age range of participants was 18 to 81 years; the mean age was 38.63 years (S.D. = 11.74). See Table 1 for demographic information. The majority of the sample was white. Participants in this study were well educated, with most respondents completing a college or graduate degree or attaining some college education. The majority of the participants worked full-time. A large number of the respondents (*n* = 174, 15.4%) checked more than one response related to work status. For example, the participant could be retired yet working part-time. A majority of the respondents identified professional occupations, and the majority of the women reported middle class status. However, the mean annual income for the sample was $33,932.59 (S.D. = $21,646.13). Most of the women lived in a city while a small number of participants resided in rural areas. Almost half of the participants lived with a female sexual partner; yet 21% lived alone. Twenty-five percent of the sample had been married to man. A large number of the women indicated that they had no faith-based affiliations. The most prominent religious affiliation was Unitarian.

Participants were asked about personal and family history of cancer. Fifty-five (4.8%) women indicated that they had had cancer. The mean age for cancer diagnosis was 39.5 (S.D. = 12.04) years, with an age range of 16 to 70 years. Biological family history of cancer was reported for 713 (62.7%) women. Of those reporting cancer in specific family members, mothers (*n* = 116; 27.8%), fathers (*n* = 77; 18.5%), and maternal grandmothers (*n* = 71; 17%) were most often listed. When participants (N = 1139) were asked about the cause of death of immediate biological family members (parents, siblings, children), 5.9% of mothers (*n* = 67) and 7.7% of fathers (*n* = 88) had died of cancer. Cancer deaths were also reported in siblings (sisters: *n* = 4; 0.4%; brothers: *n* = 14; 1.3%) and children (daughters: *n* = 1; 0.1%; sons: *n* = 3; 0.3%).

### Cancer Prevention Patterns

*Smoking:* ACS recommends that all smokers quit smoking (ACS, 2005). Most participants in this study did not smoke (n = 914; 81.7%) (Table 2). Those who did smoke (*n* = 205; 18.3%) smoked an average of 14.47 (S.D. = 9.75) cigarettes per day; range: 1-50 cigarettes/day. Participants smoked an average of 14.56 years (S.D. = 11.29); range of 1 to 60 years. Other participants reported a history of smoking. These 368 women quit smoking an average of 11.2 years ago (S.D. = 9.82; range = .01-56 years).

*Nutrition:* General ACS guidelines for nutrition include eating plenty of fruits, vegetables and whole grain foods and limiting intake of red meats and high fat foods (ACS, 2005). Participants in this study ate on

TABLE 1. Demographic Information

| Variable | n | % |
|---|---|---|
| Education [n = 1136] | | |
|     Less than high school | 17 | 1.5 |
|     High school | 24 | 2.1 |
|     Vocational training | 14 | 1.2 |
|     Some college | 229 | 20.2 |
|     College | 326 | 28.7 |
|     Graduate school | 509 | 44.8 |
|     Other | 17 | 1.5 |
| Employment [n = 1132] | | |
|     Student | 70 | 6.2 |
|     Unemployed | 41 | 3.6 |
|     Employed part-time | 108 | 9.5 |
|     Employed full-time | 683 | 60.3 |
|     Retired | 51 | 4.5 |
|     Disabled | 5 | .4 |
|     Individuals reporting multiple responses | 174 | 15.4 |
| Occupation [n = 291] | | |
|     Unskilled | 34 | 11.7 |
|     Clerical | 12 | 4.1 |
|     Skilled | 29 | 10.0 |
|     Sales | 3 | 1.0 |
|     Professional | 172 | 59.1 |
|     Middle management | 21 | 7.2 |
|     Unemployed/retired/student | 20 | 6.9 |
| Class Identity [n = 1079] | | |
|     Poor | 100 | 9.3 |
|     Working class | 315 | 29.2 |
|     Middle class | 548 | 50.8 |
|     Upper class | 99 | 9.2 |
|     Other | 17 | 1.6 |
| Race [n = 1131] | | |
|     Asian | 8 | .8 |
|     Black | 46 | 4.1 |
|     Hispanic | 20 | 1.8 |
|     Jewish | 30 | 2.7 |
|     White | 848 | 75.0 |
|     Other ethnic | 42 | 3.8 |
|     Mixed ethnic | 137 | 12.1 |
| Living in a: [n = 1123] | | |
|     City | 644 | 57.3 |
|     Suburb | 277 | 24.7 |
|     Rural area | 162 | 14.4 |
|     Other | 40 | 3.6 |

| Variable | n | % |
|---|---|---|
| Religion [n = 1086] | | |
| Catholic | 98 | 9.0 |
| Jewish | 92 | 8.5 |
| Protestant | 140 | 12.9 |
| Unitarian | 301 | 27.7 |
| None | 346 | 32.0 |
| Other | 108 | 9.9 |
| Persons living in household: | | |
| Female sexual partner [n = 1137] | 558 | 49.1 |
| Female roommate [n = 1136] | 166 | 14.6 |
| Male sexual partner [n = 1136] | 7 | .6 |
| Male roommate [n = 1136] | 63 | 5.5 |
| Your children [n = 1137] | 92 | 8.1 |
| Partner's children [n = 1136] | 42 | 3.7 |
| Roommate's children [n = 1136] | 8 | .7 |
| Your parents [n = 1136] | 44 | 3.9 |
| No one [n = 1137] | 239 | 21.0 |
| Other [n = 1136] | 82 | 7.2 |
| History of relationship with a man | | |
| Married [n = 1065] | 265 | 24.9 |
| Divorced [n = 1021] | 218 | 21.4 |
| Widowed [n = 904] | 16 | 1.8 |
| Separated [n = 919] | 68 | 7.4 |

the average 2.13 (S.D. = 1.42) servings of fruit per day and 2.60 (S.D. = 1.48) servings of vegetables per day. The women reported an intake of 3.3 (S.D. = 1.53) servings of starches and grains per day. Approximately a third of the sample (n = 345; 30.3%) indicated that they regularly ate a diet high in fiber and bran. At the other extreme, 30.8% (n = 351) indicated that they never or rarely ate foods high in fiber and bran (Table 3).

The average servings of meats consumed per week was 1.66 (S.D. = 1.85). Interestingly, 36.2% (n = 401) of the women ate no meat. Chicken or turkey was consumed more often, averaging 2.27 (S.D. = 1.76) servings per week. Many women indicated that they did not eat fish or seafood (n = 420; 38.5%). The average weekly servings of fish and seafood reported by respondents was 1.8 servings per week (S.D. = 2.29). Participants were asked to indicate their intake of saturated (butter, stick margarine, fried food, mayonnaise) and unsaturated (tub or squeeze bottle margarine, vegetable oil) fats. Respondents consumed an average of 1.66 (S.D. = 1.45) servings of saturated fats per day while the average consumption of unsaturated fats was 1.30 (S.D. = 1.31) servings per day (Table 3).

## TABLE 2. General Cancer Prevention Behaviors

| Prevention Behaviors | | n | % |
|---|---|---|---|
| Smoking | Do you smoke cigarettes? | | |
| | Yes | 205 | 18.3 |
| | No | 914 | 81.7 |
| Diet | How often do you make high bran or fiber a part of your diet? | | |
| | Never | 99 | 8.9 |
| | Rarely | 252 | 22.6 |
| | Sometimes | 421 | 37.7 |
| | Regularly | 345 | 30.9 |
| Exercise | Attainment of ACS exercise guideline | | |
| | Did not meet criterion | 452 | 63.0 |
| | Met criterion | 266 | 37.0 |
| Alcohol Use | How often do you take two or more alcoholic drinks per day? | | |
| | Never | 492 | 43.8 |
| | Rarely | 429 | 38.2 |
| | Sometimes | 150 | 13.3 |
| | Regularly | 53 | 4.7 |
| Safe Sex Practices | Do you practice safer sex? | | |
| | Yes | 608 | 58.6 |
| | No | 429 | 41.4 |
| Sun Screen Use | How often do you use sunscreen? | | |
| | Never | 68 | 6.0 |
| | Rarely | 159 | 14.1 |
| | Sometimes | 516 | 45.6 |
| | Regularly | 388 | 34.3 |

*Exercise:* Of the 1139 respondents, 718 (63%) women indicated that they exercised weekly. The ACS Guideline for exercise suggests that an individual gets 30-45 minutes of physical activity at least five days per week (ACS, 2005). In this study 266 (37%) individuals met or exceeded the criterion; however, 452 (63%) women reported weekly physical activity that did not reach the recommended 2-3 hours per week (Table 2). The most frequently reported exercise activities included walking, jogging, bicycling, and aerobic exercise (Table 4).

*Weight:* Maintaining a healthy weight is recommended by ACS (ACS, 2005). Data was not collected on the participants' actual weight or its relationship to their ideal body weight. However, data was at-

TABLE 3. Nutrition: Cancer Prevention Behavior

| Food Types | Servings Per Day | | | | | | | | | | | | | | | |
|---|---|---|---|---|---|---|---|---|---|---|---|---|---|---|---|---|
| | 0 | | 1 | | 2 | | 3 | | 4 | | 5 | | 6 | | 7 | |
| | n | % | n | % | n | % | n | % | n | % | n | % | n | % | n | % |
| Starches, grains | 7 | .6 | 91 | 8.2 | 263 | 23.8 | 338 | 30.5 | 188 | 17.0 | 111 | 10.0 | 53 | 4.8 | 56 | 5.1 |
| Fruit | 71 | 6.4 | 348 | 31.3 | 343 | 30.9 | 186 | 16.7 | 95 | 8.6 | 36 | 3.2 | 8 | 0.7 | 24 | 2.2 |
| Vegetables | 18 | 1.6 | 243 | 22.0 | 348 | 31.6 | 250 | 22.7 | 136 | 12.3 | 48 | 4.4 | 24 | 2.2 | 36 | 3.3 |
| Dairy Products | 85 | 7.7 | 296 | 26.8 | 290 | 26.2 | 236 | 21.4 | 105 | 9.5 | 42 | 3.8 | 22 | 2.0 | 29 | 2.6 |
| Saturated Fats | 199 | 18.2 | 409 | 37.3 | 256 | 23.4 | 133 | 12.1 | 46 | 4.2 | 18 | 1.6 | 16 | 1.5 | 19 | 1.7 |
| Unsaturated Fats | 310 | 28.6 | 415 | 38.3 | 211 | 19.4 | 84 | 7.7 | 30 | 2.8 | 18 | 1.7 | 5 | 0.5 | 12 | 1.1 |

| Food Types | Servings Per Week | | | | | | | | | | | | | | | |
|---|---|---|---|---|---|---|---|---|---|---|---|---|---|---|---|---|
| | 0 | | 1 | | 2 | | 3 | | 4 | | 5 | | 6 | | 7 | |
| | n | % | n | % | n | % | n | % | n | % | n | % | n | % | n | % |
| Beef, pork, lamb, veal | 401 | 36.2 | 238 | 21.5 | 170 | 15.3 | 128 | 11.6 | 68 | 6.1 | 49 | 4.4 | 13 | 1.2 | 41 | 3.7 |
| Chicken, turkey | 222 | 19.9 | 185 | 16.6 | 224 | 20.1 | 234 | 21.0 | 118 | 10.6 | 82 | 7.4 | 22 | 2.0 | 26 | 2.3 |
| Fish, seafood | 420 | 38.5 | 352 | 32.3 | 179 | 16.4 | 85 | 7.8 | 30 | 2.7 | 13 | 1.2 | 4 | 0.4 | 7 | 0.6 |
| Eggs | 336 | 30.6 | 391 | 35.6 | 189 | 17.2 | 90 | 8.2 | 59 | 5.4 | 20 | 1.8 | 2 | 0.2 | 10 | 0.9 |
| Tofu, dried beans, nuts | 352 | 32.1 | 245 | 22.3 | 166 | 15.1 | 128 | 11.7 | 77 | 7.0 | 51 | 4.6 | 21 | 1.9 | 57 | 5.2 |

TABLE 4. Exercise Activities and ACS Guidelines for Exercise

| Activity | Did Not Meet Criterion | | Met or Exceed Criterion | |
|---|---|---|---|---|
| | n | % | n | % |
| Walking/hiking outdoors | 132 | 50.4 | 130 | 49.6 |
| Jogging slower than 10 min/mile | 85 | 88.5 | 11 | 11.5 |
| Running 10 minute mile or faster | 41 | 78.8 | 11 | 21.2 |
| Bicycling | 98 | 73.7 | 35 | 26.3 |
| Aerobic exercise | 155 | 69.1 | 69 | 30.9 |
| Tennis/squash/racquetball | 31 | 93.9 | 2 | 6.1 |
| Lap swimming | 30 | 78.9 | 8 | 21.1 |

tained on weight gain and loss patterns. The respondents were asked to report the difference between their highest and lowest weight (excluding illness and pregnancy) over the last two years. Fluctuations in weight were reported by 1084 (96%) women. In light of natural metabolic changes associated with age, fluctuations in weight were examined by age groups (less than 40 years; $\geq$ 40 years). In women less than 40 years of age, 224 (38.2%) gained or lost 2-9 pounds over two years, while 284 (48.6) saw weight fluctuations of 10-29 pounds in the same time frame. Seventy-seven women ($n$ = 77, 13.2%) reported weight changes of more than 30 pounds in two years. In women 40 years and older, 207 (44.8%) gained or lost 2-9 pounds in two years. Weight fluctuations of 10-29 pounds were reported by 207 (44.8%) participants, while 48 (10.4%) women indicated weight changes of greater than 30 pounds. Information about methods for weight management was requested. The most common methods reported were exercise ($n$ = 721), low fat diet ($n$ = 459), and calorie restriction ($n$ = 333).

Over a two-year period, unintentional weight loss (e.g., due to illness, unusual stress, depression) was reported by 321 (28.4%) women. Unintentional weight loss was relatively minimal for 137 (43.1%) respondents reporting weight loss. However, 157 (49.3%) lesbians lost between 10-29 pounds over two years. Twenty-four lesbians (7.5%) lost more than 30 pounds over a two-year period.

*Alcohol Use:* ACS recommends limiting alcohol intake to one alcoholic drink per day (ACS, 2005). The majority of participants ($n$ = 808, 71.6%) reported drinking alcohol (Table 5). Preferred alcoholic bever-

TABLE 5. Alcohol Use Among Lesbians

| Item | Yes | | No | |
|------|-----|-----|-----|-----|
| | *n* | % | *n* | % |
| Do you drink alcohol? (Beer, wine, liquors) | 808 | 71.6 | 321 | 28.4 |
| Do you believe that you are a normal drinker? | 705 | 72.4 | 269 | 27.6 |
| Does anyone close to you worry or complain about your drinking? | 69 | 6.9 | 934 | 93.1 |
| Do you have or have you ever had alcoholism? | 139 | 12.2 | 998 | 87.8 |
| Are you in recovery for alcoholism? | 121 | 24.6 | 370 | 75.4 |

ages were wine/beer ($n$ = 519, 45.7%) and liquors ($n$ = 290, 25.5%). When asked how often they drank two or more drinks per day, 82% ($n$ = 921) indicated that they never/rarely consumed two or more drinks a day; 13.3% ($n$ = 150) indicated that they sometimes have two or more drinks per day, while 4.7% ($n$ = 53) reported drinking that quantity daily. Respondents who reported drinking on a weekly basis consumed an average of 4.14 (SD = 4.9) drinks per week. The range of drinks consumed per week was 1-38 while the median was two drinks per week and the mode was 1 drink per week. When asked whether they perceived themselves to be a normal drinker, 269 (27.6%) responded "no" while 705 (72.4%) believed their drinking patterns were "normal." When asked whether anyone close to them complained or worried about their drinking behaviors, 69 (6.9%) gave a positive response.

Of those indicating that they do not drink alcohol ($n$ = 321, 28.4%), 139 (12.2%) women reported a history of alcoholism. Of these, 121 (24.6%) stated that they were in recovery for alcoholism.

*Hormone Replacement:* ACS suggests discussing the benefits and risks of HRT and the use of oral contraceptives with one's health care provider (ACS, 2005). One hundred eighty-one women ($n$ = 181) indicated they had or were taking HRT for an average of 7.74 (SD = 4.61) years duration. The range of years on HRT was 1 month to 30 years; the median and mode were both 9 years.

*Safe Sex Practices:* The majority of women ($n$ = 608, 58.6%) reported practicing safe sex (Table 2). According to ACS, practicing safer sex includes using barrier protection each time an individual has sex (ACS, 2005). Three hundred seventy-two ($n$ = 372, 48.8%) women indicated they almost always/always used safe sex practices; 108 (11.3%) respondents sometimes used safe sex precautions; 50 (5.2%) women rarely used safe sex practices. The remainder (*n* = 430, 44.8%) never practiced safe sex. Safe sex practices used by these women are listed in rank order: monogamy/single partner (*n* = 439); sex with known women (*n* = 253); mutual masturbation (*n* = 209); massage (*n* = 194); latex gloves and finger cots (*n* = 138); dental dams (*n* = 115). Other safe sex practices listed included: use of vaginal condoms (n = 80); sex with known men (*n* = 32); monogamy/single partner sex (*n* = 30); mutual masturbation (*n* = 28); condoms for oral sex (*n* = 23).

*Sunscreen Use:* Using sunscreen with an SPF of 15 or higher and reapplying often is recommended by ACS (ACS, 2005). Skin protection with sunscreen use was examined. Sixty-eight women (*n* = 68; 6%) never used sunscreen; 159 (14.1%) rarely used sunscreen protection. Almost half of the women (*n* = 516, 45.6%) sometimes used sunscreen, while 388 (34.3%) regularly safeguarded their skin from the sun.

### Screening Patterns

*Breast Health:* ACS guidelines for breast screening for women ages 20-39 years include a monthly SBE and a clinical breast exam by a health care professional every three years (Smith, Cokkinides & Eyre, 2003). Although 192 (16.9%) women reported a history of breast problems, only 9.4% (*n* = 55) of the women in this age group conducted monthly SBE. Of major concern is the fact that 17.8% (*n* = 104) of the women had never done SBE (Table 6). The majority of the women in this age group (*n* = 494; 84.6%) were likely to have had a breast exam by a health care provider within the last 3 years. The clinical breast examination by the provider was most often done during an office visit for a physical examination (*n* = 440; 82.7%). Although the ACS guidelines do not recommend mammogram screening for women ages 20-39, 109 (18.7%) of these participants had had a mammogram.

Breast health screening recommendations for women age 40 and above include a yearly mammogram, a yearly CBE by a health care professional, and a SBE every month (Smith, Cokkinides & Eyre, 2003). A majority of the lesbians (*n* = 277; 57.1%) in this age category reported having a mammogram within the last year; however, almost ten percent (*n* = 47) indicated that they had never had mammogram. Adherence to the ACS standard for breast exams conducted by a provider was high; 378 (77.6%) stated that they had had a clinical breast exam within the last year. Only 2 (0.4%) participants had never been examined by a provider. In most cases the clinical breast exam occurred during a physical examination (*n* = 308; 67.7%). Only 15% (*n* = 73) conducted SBE on a

TABLE 6. Breast Health Screening Patterns of Lesbians

| Variable | Ages 20-39 | | Ages 40 and above | |
|---|---|---|---|---|
| | *n* | % | *n* | % |
| Frequency of SBE | N = 584 | | N = 488 | |
| Never | 104 | 17.8 | 65 | 13.3 |
| Less than 3 times/year | 177 | 30.3 | 109 | 22.3 |
| 3-4/year | 148 | 25.3 | 135 | 27.7 |
| Every other month | 84 | 14.4 | 84 | 17.2 |
| Once a month | 55 | 9.4 | 73 | 15.0 |
| Two times/month | 16 | 2.7 | 22 | 4.5 |
| Last Mammogram | N = 584 | | N = 485 | |
| Never | 475 | 81.3 | 47 | 9.7 |
| More than 5 years ago | 25 | 4.3 | 25 | 5.2 |
| Within last 5 years | 15 | 2.6 | 31 | 6.4 |
| Within last 3 years | 13 | 2.2 | 31 | 6.4 |
| Within last 2 years | 18 | 3.1 | 74 | 15.3 |
| Within last year | 38 | 6.5 | 277 | 57.1 |
| Last Breast Exam by Provider | N = 584 | | N = 487 | |
| Never | 31 | 5.3 | 2 | 0.4 |
| More than 5 years ago | 23 | 3.9 | 16 | 3.3 |
| Within last 5 years | 36 | 6.2 | 17 | 3.5 |
| Within last 3 years | 34 | 5.8 | 25 | 5.1 |
| Within last 2 years | 84 | 14.4 | 49 | 10.1 |
| Within last year | 376 | 64.4 | 378 | 77.6 |
| Circumstances of last Breast Exam (N = 532) | N = 532 | | N = 455 | |
| With visit for mammogram | 12 | 2.3 | 58 | 12.7 |
| With physical exam | 440 | 82.7 | 308 | 67.7 |
| Request during routine office visit | 19 | 3.6 | 16 | 3.5 |
| Appointment specifically for breast exam | 61 | 11.5 | 73 | 16.0 |

monthly basis; nearly as many (13.3%, *n* = 65) had never performed a SBE.

*Gynecological Health:* Many of the lesbians (*n* = 295; 25.9%) responding to this survey reported gynecological problems. The majority of the participants (52.9%, *n* = 597) reported having an annual PAP smear. At the other extreme, 64 (5.7%) had never had a PAP smear and 64 (5.7%) indicated that it had been more than 5 years between gynecological examinations (Table 7). This is of concern as 890 (79.6%) participants reported having had an abnormal PAP smear.

Although data were not collected on initiation of sexual activity or the type of cervical cancer screening tests, screening practices by age will be reported. Of the 38 women ages 20 years or younger, 19 (50%) had never had a PAP smear. Eight (21.1%) lesbians had annual cervical

TABLE 7. Gynecological Screening Patterns by Age

| Frequency of PAP Smear | Ages < 20 | | Ages 21-30 | | Ages 31-70 | |
|---|---|---|---|---|---|---|
| | n | % | n | % | n | % |
| | N = 38 | | N = 273 | | N = 769 | |
| Never | 19 | 50 | 21 | 7.7 | 19 | 2.5 |
| More than every 5 years | 1 | 2.6 | 18 | 6.6 | 42 | 5.5 |
| Every 3 to 5 years | 2 | 5.3 | 28 | 10.3 | 113 | 14.7 |
| Once every 2 years | 4 | 10.5 | 55 | 20.1 | 142 | 18.5 |
| Once a year | 8 | 21.1 | 138 | 50.5 | 427 | 55.5 |
| Every 3 to 6 months | 4 | 10.5 | 13 | 4.8 | 26 | 3.4 |

Note: Data for women > 70 is not included in this table.

screening. Depending on the type of cytology testing used, women in the 21-30 year age group should be having annual or biannual PAP smears (ACS, 2003). In this sample, 206 (75.4%) of the respondents followed the ACS Guidelines for Cervical Cancer Screening (ACS, 2003). Twenty-one women (7.7%, $n = 21$) in the 21-30 year age group had never had a PAP smear. Screening recommendations for women ages 31-70 years indicate that screening every 2-3 years is adequate if no abnormal cytology tests occur for three consecutive screenings (ACS, 2003). The majority of women in this age group ($n = 595$; 77.4%) met these guidelines. Nineteen ($n = 19$, 2.5%) of the women in the 31-70 year age group had never had a PAP smear. There were 11 women in this sample between the ages of 71 and 81 years of age; four (36.4%) of these women had never had a PAP smear.

## DISCUSSION

### Cancer Prevention Patterns

*Smoking:* Less than 20% of participants in this study smoked. These results are similar to the 20.1% reported in BLHP I study (Roberts & Sorensen, 1999) and comparable to the BRFSS report of women in general (20.3%). Smoking patterns in lesbians in this study are no different than women in general.

*Nutrition:* Proposed guidelines for building a better food pyramid (Harvard School of Public Health, 2004) give direction to interpreting these findings. New guidelines suggest that vegetables should be eaten in abundance, women in this study ate 2.6 servings of vegetables per day. Intake of fruits was 2.13 servings per day, thus these women met the guidelines of 2-3 servings of fruit per day. Lesbians in this study reported an intake of 3.3 servings of starches and grains per day. New guidelines suggest that all starches should be consumed sparingly. Approximately a third of this sample reported eating a diet high in fiber and bran suggesting that these lesbians may meet the new guidelines by eating whole grain foods at most meals. However, approximately 70% did not consume high fiber diets.

Participants consumed 2.2 servings of chicken or turkey per week and average weekly servings of fish and seafood were 1.8 servings per week. New nutrition guidelines (Harvard School of Public Health, 2004) indicate that fish, poultry and eggs should be eaten 0-2 times per day. On the average women in this study consumed approximately 4 servings of chicken/turkey and fish/seafood per week, meeting the proposed guidelines. Red meat is to be consumed sparingly. Women averaged 1.6 servings of red meat per week, however, 36.2% of the women ate no meat. Respondents consumed an average of 1.66 servings of saturated fats per day; guidelines suggest that butter and saturated fats be used sparingly.

*Exercise:* ACS guidelines suggest that individuals get 30 minutes of exercise most days (ACS, 2005). In this study only 30% of the women met or exceeded this criterion, while 63% reported weekly physical activity that did not reach the recommended 2-3 hours per week. In the Nurses' Health Study II, lesbians (75.9%) were slightly more likely to exercise than heterosexual women (69.3%), with 10% more lesbians reporting strenuous exercise once a week or more (Case, Austin, Hunter, Manson, Malspeis, Willett & Spiegelman, 2004). Although exercise was measured differently in both studies, lesbians may exercise more than their heterosexual counterparts.

*Weight:* Results in this study indicate that weight fluctuations among these women were common. ACS Guidelines suggest that achieving and maintaining a healthy weight is important (ACS, 2005). In the Nurses' Health Study II, 21.3% of the lesbians reported a 10 pound weight gain over three years while only 14.6% of the heterosexuals gained this amount (Case et al., 2004). Both studies suggest that lesbians do not maintain a consistent weight. Weight management strategies that foster weight loss and maintenance are recommended for this population.

*Alcohol Use:* Results from studies about alcohol use among lesbians are difficult to interpret. Many studies only report that lesbians consumed alcohol but did not describe consumption patterns. In this study, 71% of the women reported drinking alcohol while 57.5% reported alcohol use in a study by Aaron and colleagues (2001). Robertson and Sorensen (1999) noted that 24.4% of their respondents reported drinking 2 or more drinks per day sometimes/regularly. In contrast, this study found that only 13.3% indicated that they sometimes drink two or more drinks per day. The majority of the women (72.4%) believed that their drinking patterns were normal; however, for those women (4.7%) who drank two or more drinks daily and those whose families/friends were concerned about their drinking behaviors (6.9%), support for decreased consumption is recommended. Guidelines for alcohol use suggest moderate consumption of alcohol. The U.S. Department of Agriculture's *Nutrition & Your Health* publication (2000) advises that women should limit their alcohol intake to one drink per day. Using this guideline as a marker, 82% of the lesbians in this study would probably meet this marker as they indicated that they never/rarely consumed two or more drinks a day.

*Safe Sex Practices:* Reports of safe sex practices among lesbians are variable and not easily comparable across studies. For example, Diamont et al. (2000) reported that 89% of participants engaged in vaginal intercourse without a condom and Carroll et al. (1997) noted that a lack of protection was reported by 34% of the women experiencing penile-vaginal penetration and 40.6% engaging in penile-anal penetration. Women in this study described a broader array of sexual behaviors with 58.6% of the women reporting practicing safe sex suggesting that more lesbians in this sample practiced safe sex than reported in some studies.

*Sunscreen Use:* In studies that included men and women, Johnson and Lookingbill (1984) reported sunscreen use by 41% of their sample, while Prium et al. (1999) reported that 76% of their sample used sunscreen and 61% reported reapplying it. In our study lesbians (79.9%) sometimes/regularly used sunscreen. These lesbians reported higher income and education levels which supports Purdue's findings (2002) that individuals with higher income and educational levels were likely to use sunscreen. Clearly the use of sunscreen has increased since the 1984 Johnson and Lookingbill study. However, the estimated numbers of new cases of melanoma and other skin cancers continue to increase (59,350 individuals in 2004 [Jemal, Tiwari, Murray, Ghafoor, Samuels, Ward, Feuer, & Thun, 2004]), reinforcing the need for consistent use of sunscreen by those exposed to sun via work or social activities.

## Screening Patterns

*Breast Health:* SBE practices are very useful in locating breast cysts yet self breast exams were used sparingly among women in this sample.

Although the majority of the lesbians ages 20-39 years did have a CBE every three years as recommended (Smith, Cokkinides & Eyre, 2003), very few performed monthly SBE. Regular SBE are critical to assure no breast nodules develop in this three year span. By age 40, the risk for being diagnosed with breast cancer is 1 in 235. While breast cancer is less common at a younger age, young women tend to have a more aggressive disease. Like the younger cohort, lesbians age 40 years and older were not likely to conduct SBE on a regular basis. Although the majority of these women had an annual mammogram (57.1%) and/or a CBE (77.6%), they did not recognize the value of SBE. These results suggest that SBE educational programs are warranted for lesbians across all age groups.

Our results suggest that older women who have higher incomes and who regularly have physical exams and perform SBE are more likely to have regular mammograms. Similarly, Rankow and Tessaro (1998) found that older lesbians with higher incomes and insurance were more likely to have a mammogram. Access to mammography screening should be made available to all women. Research should explore factors that prevent lesbians and heterosexual women from having regular mammograms. In addition, age-specific strategies to encourage adherence to the ACS guidelines need to be developed and tested.

*Gynecological Health: Cervical Cancer Screening.* Although 75.4% of the women ages 21-30 had annual cervical screenings, about one fourth of them did not follow ACS guidelines (ACS, 2003), placing them at risk for undiagnosed cervical dysplasia or cancer. The majority of women ages 31-70 years met the ACS Guidelines for Cervical Cancer Screening (ACS, 2003), yet one fourth of these women did not follow the guidelines. As noted, a large number of these lesbians (79.6%) reported abnormal PAP smears, possibly putting them at higher risk for cervical cancer or other gynecologic problems. Clearly strategies that encourage women to follow recommended cervical cancer screening guidelines are warranted. Again these strategies should be age-specific.

*Limitations:* Use of a convenience sample limited the generalizability of the present results, since volunteer samples tend to have better health behaviors than representative samples of the population. In addition, response bias may have further limited the study as participants may have given socially desirable responses concerning their health behaviors on the surveys. Having no specified comparison group further inhibits the interpretation of the results. All lesbians did not have access to participation in the study even though sampling methods were diverse and widespread. In spite of these limitations, the results of this replication study provide a better understanding of lesbian health patterns related to cancer prevention and screening. In addition, knowledge about the profile of lesbians most likely to obtain a mammogram gives direction to research for improving mammogram screening rates among younger, less affluent lesbians. Also an understanding of the eating and exercise patterns of lesbians supports the development of interventions to improve nutrition, weight management, and exercise participation, thus assuring healthier lifestyles among lesbians.

## IMPLICATIONS FOR PRACTICE AND RESEARCH

- Educational interventions based on the "new" nutrition pyramid would be helpful with emphasis on increasing fiber and decreasing starches and saturated fats in the diet of lesbians. Weight loss and maintenance strategies should also be included.
- Interventions to encourage appropriate and regular exercise activities need to be identified and tested to assure an active lifestyle over time.
- Safe sex practices used by this sample were varied. Further research efforts that establish reasonable guidelines for safe sex practices among lesbians are needed.
- Although the use of sunscreen has increased, media campaigns to encourage skin protection among all age groups would help to decrease the incidence of skin cancer.
- Strategies that educate lesbians of all ages, ethnic groups, and cultures about the value of and method for SBE need to be identified and tested.

In general, lesbians in this sample met most of the ACS cancer prevention and screening guidelines (ACS, 2003; ACS, 2005; Smith, Cokkinides & Eyre, 2003). Areas for improvement of behaviors were nutrition, weight management, exercise, safer sex practices, sunscreen use and self-breast examination. Interventions to foster adherence to the ACS Guidelines in these areas are warranted.

## REFERENCES

Aaron, D. J., Markovic, N., Danielson, M.E., Honnold, J. A., Janosky, J.E., & Schmidt, N.J. (2001). Behaviorial risk factors for disease and preventive health practices among lesbians. *American Journal of Public Health, 91*(6), 972-975.

American Cancer Society (2003). Screening guidelines for the early detection of cancer in asymptomatic people. In *Cancer Prevention and Early Detection, Facts and Figures.* Atlanta, Georgia: American Cancer Society.

American Cancer Society (2005). Cancer prevention and early detection workshop for women. Retrieved on September 28, 2005 from http://www.cancer.org/downloads/PED/cancer%20Prevention%20and%20Early%20Detection%20Worksheet%20for%20Women.pdf.

Bradford, J., Ryan, C., & Rothblum, E. D. (1994). National lesbian health care survey: Implications for mental health care. *Journal of Consulting & Clinical Psychology* 62(2), 228-242.

Bradford, J., & Ryan, C. (1988). *The National Lesbian Health Care Survey.* Washington, DC: National Lesbian and Gay Health Foundation.

Burnett, C.B., Steakley, C.S., Slack, R., Roth, J., & Lerman, C. (1999). Patterns of breast cancer screening among lesbians at increased risk for breast cancer. *Women and Health*, 29(4), 35-55.

Carroll, N., Goldstein, R. S., Lo, W., & Mayer, K. H. (1997). Gynecological infections and sexual practices of Massachusetts lesbian and bisexual women. *Journal of the Gay and Lesbian Medical Association* 1(1), 15-23.

Case, P., Austin, S. B., Hunter, D. J., Manson, J. E., Malspeis, S., Willett, W. C., & Spiegelman, D. (2004). Sexual orientation, health risks factors, and physical functioning in the Nurses' Health Study II. *Journal of Women's Health*, 13(9), 1033-1047.

Cochran, S. D., Mays, V. M., Bowen, D., Gage, S., Bybee, D., Roberts, S. J., Goldstein, R.S., Robison, A., Rankow, E.J., & White, J. (2001). Cancer-related risk indicators and preventive screening behaviors among lesbians and bisexual women. *American Journal of Public Health*, 91(4), 591-597.

Diamant, A. L., Schuster, M. A., & Lever, J. (2000). Receipt of preventive health care services by lesbians. *American Journal of Preventive Medicine*, 19(3), 141-148.

Dibble, S. L., Roberts, S. A., Robertson, P. A., & Paul, S. M. (2002). *Oncology Nursing Forum* 29 (1), 29. Retrieved on April 18, 2004 from www.ons.org/xp6/ONS/Library.xml/ONS_Publications.xml/ONF.xml/ONF2002.xml/Jan_Feb_2002.xml

Fishman, S. J. & Anderson, E. H. (2003). Perception of HIV and safer sexual behaviors among lesbians. *Journal of the Association of Nurses in AIDS Care*, 14(6), 48-55.

Greene, A. L., Torio, C. M., & Klassen, A. C. (2005). Measuring sustained mammography use by urban African American women. *Journal of Community Health*, 30(4), 235-251.

Harvard School of Public Health. (2004). Food Pyramids: Nutrition Source. Retrieved on September 22, 2005 from http://www.hsph.harvard.edu/nutritionsource/pyramids.html.

Hughes, T. L., & Jacobson, K. M. (2003). Sexual orientation and women's smoking. *Current Women's Health Report* 3(3), 254-61.

Jemal, A., Tiwari, R. C., Murray, T., Ghafoor, A., Samuels, A., Ward, E., Feuer, E. J., & Thun, M. J. (2004). Cancer Statistics, 2004. *CA, A Cancer Journal for Clinicians*, 54 (1), 8-29.

Johnson, E. Y., & Lookingbill, D. P. (1984). Sunscreen use and sun exposure. Trends in a white population. *Archive of Dermatology* 120(6), 727-731.

Johnson, S. R., Guenther, S. M., Laube, D. W., & Keetel, W.C. (1981). Factors influencing lesbian gynecological care: A preliminary study. *American Journal of Obstetrics and Gynecology*, 27(3), 724-730.

Johnson, S. R., Smith, E. M., & Guenther, S. M. (1987). Comparison of gynecological health care problems between lesbian and bisexual women. *The Journal of Reproductive Medicine, 32*(11), 805-811.

Koh, A. S. (2000). Use of preventive health behaviors by lesbian, bisexual, and heterosexual women: questionnaire survey. *Western Journal of Medicine 172*(6), 379-384.

Lairson, D. R., Chan, W., & Newmark, G. R. (2005). Determinants of the demand for breast cancer screening among women veterans in the United States. *Social Science and Medicine, 61*(7), 1608-1617.

Lauver, D. R., Karon, S. L., Egan, J., Jacobson, M., Nugent, J., Settersten, L., & Shaw, V. (1999). Understanding lesbians' mammography utilization. *Women's Health Issues 9*(5), 264-274.

Munro, Barbara H. (2005). *Statistical Methods for Health Care Research*, 5th edition, Philadelphia, PA: Lippincott, Williams and Wilkins. Ch. 13.

National Center for Health Statistics. (2004). Health, United States, 2004, with Chartbook on Trends in the Health of Americans. Hyattsville, MD: National Center for Health Statistics. Retrieved September 22, 2005, from http://www.cdc.gov/nchs/data/hus/hus04trend.pdf#081

Nutrition and Your Health: Dietary Guidelines for Americans. (2000). Fifth edition: U.S. Department of Agriculture, U.S. Department of Health and Human Services, 36-37.

Pruim, D., Wright, L., & Green, A. (1999) Do people who apply sunscreens, re-apply them? *Australian Journal of Dermatology 40*(2), 79-82.

Purdue, M. P. (2002) Predictors of sun protection in Canadian adults. *Canadian Journal of Public Health 93*(6), 470-474.

Rankow, E. J., & Tessaro, I. (1998). Cervical cancer risk and Papanicolaou screening in a sample of lesbian and bisexual women. *The Journal of Family Practice, 47*(2), 139-143.

Roberts, S. A., Dibble, S. L., Scanlon, J. L., Paul, S. M., & Davids, H. (1998). Differences in risk factors for breast cancer: Lesbian and heterosexual women. *Journal of the Gay and Lesbian Medical Association 2*(3), 93-101.

Roberts, S. J., & Sorensen, L. (1999). Health related behaviors and cancer screening of lesbians: Results from the Boston Lesbian Health Project. *Women & Health, 28*(4), 1-12.

Robinson, J. K., Rigel, D. S., & Amonette, R. A. (1997). Trends in sun exposure knowledge, attitudes, and behaviors: 1986 to 1996. *Journal of the American Academy of Dermatology 37*(2 Pt 1), 179-186.

Smith, R. A., Cokkinides, V., & Eyre, H. J. (2003). American Cancer Society Guidelines for the Early Detection of Cancer, 2003. *CA, A Cancer Journal for Clinicians, 53*(1), 27-43.

SPSS, Inc. (2002). SPSS 11.5 for Windows. Chicago, IL: SPSS, Inc.

Valanis, B. G., Bowen, D. J., Bassford, T., Whitlock, E., Charney, P., & Carter, R. A. (2000). Sexual orientation and health: Comparisons in the Women's Health Initiative sample. *Archives of Family Medicine, 9*(9), 843-853.

Vital and Health Statistics: Health Promotion and Disease Prevention United States 1990. Series 10: Data from the National Health Survey No. 185. Hyattsville, MD: U.S. Dept. of Health and Human Services, April 1993. [DHHS Publication No. (PHS) 93-1513].

White, J. C. & Dull, V. T. (1997). Health risk factors and health-seeking behavior in lesbians. *Journal of Women's Health, 6*(1), 103-112.

doi:10.1300/J013v44n02_02

# Sexual Minority Women's Interactions with Breast Cancer Providers

Ulrike Boehmer, PhD
Patricia Case, ScD

**SUMMARY.** Good patient-physician relationships and communication lead to better patient health and more satisfied patients. So far, satisfaction of sexual minority (lesbian, bisexual or women who partner with women) cancer patient-physician interactions is unknown. This study describes sexual minorities' experiences with their treating physicians and which provider attitudes were perceived as positive or negative. We conducted separate individual interviews with 39 sexual minority women diagnosed with breast cancer. All interviews were audio-recorded, transcribed and then analyzed from a Grounded Theory perspective. Partici-

Ulrike Boehmer is affiliated with the Boston University, School of Public Health, Department of Health Services, Boston, MA, and the Center for Health Quality, Outcomes and Economic Research (CHQOER), Bedford, MA.

Patricia Case is affiliated with the Harvard Medical School, Department of Social Medicine, and The Fenway Institute, Fenway Community Health, Boston, MA.

Address correspondence to: Ulrike Boehmer, PhD, CHQOER, 200 Springs Road (152), Bedford, MA 01730 (E-mail: boehmer@bu.edu).

The authors are grateful to the participants who shared their thoughts and experiences.

Support for this research was provided by the Susan G. Komen Breast Cancer Foundation, Grant # POP0100158, PI: U. Boehmer. Institutional support and work space for the research was provided by the Department of Veterans Affairs, Edith Nourse Rogers Memorial Veterans Hospital, Bedford, MA.

The views expressed in this article are those of the authors and do not necessarily represent the views of the Susan G. Komen Breast Cancer Foundation or the Department of Veterans Affairs.

[Haworth co-indexing entry note]: "Sexual Minority Women's Interactions with Breast Cancer Providers." Boehmer, Ulrike, and Patricia Case. Co-published simultaneously in *Women & Health* (The Haworth Medical Press, an imprint of The Haworth Press, Inc.) Vol. 44, No. 2, 2006, pp. 41-58; and: *Preventive Health Measures for Lesbian and Bisexual Women* (ed: Shelly Kerr, and Robin Mathy) The Haworth Medical Press, an imprint of The Haworth Press, Inc., 2006, pp. 41-58. Single or multiple copies of this article are available for a fee from The Haworth Document Delivery Service [1-800-HAWORTH, 9:00 a.m. - 5:00 p.m. (EST). E-mail address: docdelivery@haworthpress.com].

pants' narratives indicated that satisfaction is connected with a certain style of patient-physician interactions rather than physician gender. Specific provider traits in the two domains of (1) inter-personal behaviors and (2) medical expertise and decision-making determined patient satisfaction. These findings suggest that physicians of either gender can develop the skills needed to improve quality of breast cancer care for sexual minority women. doi:10.1300/J013v44n02_03 *[Article copies available for a fee from The Haworth Document Delivery Service: 1-800-HAWORTH. E-mail address: <docdelivery@haworthpress.com> Website: <http://www. HaworthPress.com> © 2006 by The Haworth Press, Inc. All rights reserved.]*

**KEYWORDS.** Physician-patient relations, patient satisfaction, homosexuality, female, interviews, physician's practice patterns, decision making, sex factors

## *INTRODUCTION*

Good patient-physician relationships and communication are likely to lead to positive outcomes, including higher patient satisfaction (Ong et al., 1995; Roter et al., 1997; Stewart, 1995). Aspects of physician communication that have been linked to satisfaction consist of information-giving, affective behavior (e.g., eye contact), discussing psychosocial content, and patient-centered behavior (e.g., responding to patients' ideas) (Bertakis, 1977; Bertakis et al., 1991; Hall et al., 1994; Henbest & Stewart, 1990; Ong et al., 1995). While most studies focus on satisfaction, evidence is growing that good patient-physician communication and relationships affect patients' emotional and physical health and other outcomes, such as decision-making and compliance (Beck et al., 2002; Stewart et al., 2000; Stewart, 1995). Particularly in oncology, communication is recognized as an important clinical skill, and studies have linked good communication to greater cancer-related self-efficacy and better adjustment (Baile & Aaron, 2005; Fallowfield & Jenkins, 1999; Roberts et al., 1994; Zachariae et al., 2003). Aspects of physician interactions, such as interpersonal communication, information exchange, and engaging patients in decision-making, are linked to positive outcomes (Arora, 2003; Baile & Aaron, 2005).

Researchers examined whether physician gender accounts for differences in communication and found that female physicians engage more in communication behaviors linked to positive outcomes, including satisfaction among female patients in particular (Bertakis et al., 2003;

Derose et al., 2001; Elstad, 1994; Hall & Roter, 1998; Roter et al., 2002). Whether the implications of physician gender and physician behaviors apply to sexual minority patients, that is, lesbians, bisexuals, and women who partner with women, is mostly unknown. From the available studies of sexual minority women in the context of primary care, it is known that most lesbians prefer female family doctors (Geddes, 1994; Lucas, 1992), have difficulty communicating with providers (Bonvicini & Perlin, 2003; White & Dull, 1998), including disclosing their sexual orientation to providers (Cochran & Mays, 1988; Klitzman & Greenberg, 2002; Lucas, 1992; Stein & Bonuck, 2001). About the interactions of sexual minority women in the context of cancer care, we have even less information. We reported on cancer providers' lack of inquiry about sexual orientation and how women decided on disclosure of their sexual orientation (Boehmer & Case, 2004), and others reported that lesbians are less satisfied with care compared to heterosexual breast cancer patients (Matthews et al., 2002).

Our intent in conducting this study was to describe sexual minorities' experiences with breast cancer care physicians. Specifically, we sought to explore our hypothesis that sexual minority women may experience either positive or negative provider-patient interactions that are unique to sexual minority women or, when similar to those reported elsewhere for heterosexual women, have differing manifestations.

## METHODS

We relied exclusively on sexual minority patients' reports of breast cancer care. Prior research indicated that patient reports are valid proxies of estimating patient-provider interactions (Kaplan et al., 1995). Qualitative methods were selected to maximize participants' freedom in framing information to reflect their viewpoint, rather than responding to researchers' preconceived notions of measurement categories. The Institutional Review Boards of both Boston University and Harvard Medical School approved this study's methods and materials.

### Sampling and Recruitment

The current qualitative retrospective study of sexual minorities with breast cancer relied on purposive sampling, meaning we focused on the population of sexual minority women and intentionally selected individuals that fit pre-defined criteria. This type of non-probability sampling has been widely used to overcome the unique challenges of recruiting members of vulnerable or "hidden" populations into research studies (Biernacki & Waldorf, 1981; Watters & Biernacki, 1989) and was well-suited for a comprehensive exploration of sexual minorities' experiences with breast cancer care. Recruitment was further enhanced through the use of "snowball" sampling where participants were asked to refer others who might be willing to participate in the study (Biernacki & Waldorf, 1981). Used optimally, peer-to-peer referral is an effective way to reduce sample bias by gaining access to the opinions of those who might not otherwise have volunteered to participate in a research study or been aware of the opportunity to do so.

All recruitment materials announced that participants would receive $20 for their participation. Recruitment activities were limited to the New England area. We used newspaper advertisements, Internet postings, and distribution of flyers to organizations, at events, and medical centers to publicize the study. To obtain a racially and ethnically diverse sample, one of our flyers explicitly stated our goal of recruiting African-American and Latina participants. Moreover, extensive efforts were made to reach African-American and Latina sexual minorities by handing the race-specified flyer to known African-American or Latina sexual minority women, distributing it to churches, organizations, and health centers with a high proportion of African-American and Latino patients, and at African-American or Latina centered events.

## Participants

Women were eligible for this study if they met three criteria: (1) sexual minority status, (2) having a diagnosis of breast cancer, and (3) sufficient fluency in English to participate in data collection. The use of an interpreter might have biased the disclosure of sensitive information. We defined sexual minority status as either stating a lesbian or bisexual sexual identity or reporting female partner choice. We included women who reported partnering with women to be inclusive of women who might feel uncomfortable embracing a lesbian or bisexual identity. Time since diagnosis and stage of breast cancer were unrestricted.

## Procedures

After signed, written consent was obtained, we conducted tape-recorded in-depth, semi-structured interviews. Interviews lasted approximately 90 minutes and were conducted at participants' homes, researchers' or participants' offices, or on the telephone. Interviews were conducted primarily by the principal investigator (Dr. Boehmer), who has extensive experience and training in qualitative methods, grounded theory, and narrative analysis. Using a topic guide developed by Dr. Boehmer for this project, and allowing for a conversational and flexible interviewing style to permit the participant to "tell her story," each participant was asked to tell about her experiences with diagnosis and treatment of breast cancer. Specific questions focused on the experiences with the treating physicians, including physician behaviors and communication styles that were particularly helpful or that were perceived as negative. A short self-administered questionnaire was used after the interview to collect information about the stage and timing of breast cancer and demographic characteristics of the participant, including age, race/ethnicity, sexual orientation, relationship status, education, employment, income, and insurance status. While providers' gender was collected from the participants, it was not possible to collect the providers' sexual orientation with any degree of reliability.

## Analysis

Summary statistics, including means or percent distribution, were calculated to describe participants' medical and demographic characteristics (see Table 1). The audio-recorded interview data were transcribed verbatim and imported into a qualitative data analysis package, Ethnograph (Qualis Research 2001, version 5). We used open coding, which is the process of developing categories of all possible themes emerging from the data, and developed a coding scheme. To check for reliability in coding, short segments of transcripts were coded by both investigators. Divergent coding between the two investigators was resolved through discussion, and both investigators coded additional segments until full consensus was reached on all codes. We used a grounded theory approach (Strauss & Corbin, 1990) in analysis. Grounded theory methodology uses an iterative approach to narrative data, which consists of identifying a pattern, developing a relational hypothesis, and then going back over the data to verify the hypothesis with the goal of developing a theory of understanding about participants' experiences. Following open coding, and reliability testing in coding, emergent themes and relational codes were identified. The analysis we present here focuses on participants' perceptions and interactions with their breast care providers, including the role of physician gender.

# RESULTS

## Sample Description

The medical and demographic characteristics of the 39 sexual minority women with breast cancer are summarized in Table 1. Of the self-reported sexual minority participants, most were white (95%), highly educated (98%), identified as lesbian (82.1%), had health insurance

TABLE 1. Characteristics of Study Participants (n = 39)

| Characteristic | Data |
|---|---|
| Age: Mean (Range) | 49.2 (26-67) |
| Race/Ethnicity % (n):  *White* | 94.9 (37) |
| *Latina* | 5.1 (2) |
| Sexual identity % (n):  *Lesbian* | 82.1 (32) |
| *Bisexual* | 15.4 (6) |
| *Other* | 2.6 (1) |
| Relationship status % (n):  *Single* | 28.2 (11) |
| *Partnered with a woman* | 69.2 (27) |
| *Other* | 2.6 (1) |
| Education % (n):  *High school* | 2.6 (1) |
| *College* | 46.2 (18) |
| *Graduate School* | 51.3 (20) |
| Employment % (n): *Full or part time* | 87.2 (34) |
| Income Range: *less than $10k-more than $100k* | |
| Supporting 1 person % (n) Mean | 79.5 (31) $36,774 |
| Supporting more than 1 person % (n) Mean | 20.5 ( 8) $71,250 |
| Have health insurance % (n) | 89.7 (35) |
| Stage of breast cancer % (n): *in situ* | 23.1 (9) |
| *I* | 33.3 (13) |
| *II* | 23.1 (9) |
| *III* | 5.1 (2) |
| *IV* | 12.8 (5) |
| *Unknown* | 2.6 (1) |
| Mean number of years since diagnosis (Range) | 5.5 (0-18) |
| Disclosed sexual orientation to any physician | 71.8 (28) |

(90%), worked for pay (87%), and were currently partnered (69%). Most (72%) reported that they had disclosed their sexual orientation to at least one of their breast cancer care providers. The majority (56%) had been diagnosed with early breast cancer, on average about five years ago.

A majority of these women reported having been treated by female physicians, in particular female surgeons (Table 2).

## *Physicians' Gender*

With an initial diagnosis of breast cancer, most women did not select physicians based on gender. Women reported feeling pressured to act fast, frequently went to the person suggested, and were most concerned about a physician's immediate availability and her or his medical expertise. However, whenever women were presented with an opportunity to choose among several female and male specialists, most women selected female over male physicians. They reasoned that their preference for a

TABLE 2. Gender of Treating Physicians (n = 39)

|  | % (n) |
|---|---|
| **Surgeon** | |
| Female | 79.5 (31) |
| Male | 17.9 (7) |
| Not applicable* | 2.6 (1) |
| **Radiologist** | |
| Female | 25.6 (10) |
| Male | 30.8 (12) |
| Missing gender/Not applicable§ | 43.6 (17) |
| **Oncologist** | |
| Female | 48.7 (19) |
| Male | 30.8 (12) |
| Missing gender/Not applicable§ | 20.5 (8) |
| Only female physicians‡ | 43.6 (17) |
| Only male physicians‡ | 10.3 (4) |
| Physicians of both genders‡ | 46.2 (18) |

* 1 woman did not receive surgery
§ Missing information on the gender of specialist and some did not receive treatment by this specialist
‡ Includes cases with missing gender information

female physician had to do with an increased comfort with women doctors, their perception of communication to be easier, an ascribed similarity of experiences as women, including sharing an understanding of the female body and being in tune with a woman's feelings. Further, female physicians were perceived as safer than male physicians in particular with respect to being protected from sexism and homophobia.

When women explained why male physicians were less desirable, they reported not understanding men, men's lives and their goals, and not having emotional connections with men. Male physicians were also less desirable because the women anticipated communication barriers. In particular, women described men as perpetuating a paternalistic medical establishment. Most women interviewed expressed dissatisfaction with male providers' paternalistic behavior:

> Will it affect my being able to have children, you know? . . . And he said, I don't think you should be worrying about that right now, whether or not you can have–you know, you're going to be able to have kids. Like, I don't think that should be a concern of yours. He was so angry, like at the questions I had just pissed him off. He wanted me to be like, "Oh, really? Oh, you think I should do that? Okay. I'll do whatever you say, Mr. Doctor Man." (Laughter.) And it really, really pissed him off. He was a jerk.

Nevertheless, male providers treated a sizable proportion of women, many who reported positive and satisfying interactions, while some women reported negative encounters with female providers. The following is just one example of positive experiences with male physicians:

> And [name] is not what you would call warm and fuzzy, but you have–he talks directly to you, he doesn't pull any punches, very direct, answers all your questions, is always available. And I've grown to like him a lot and trust him, in terms of information that he gives me, and his treatment decisions and, you know, recommendations and stuff. And you get a sense that he knows what he's doing and that he cares about you.

Sexual minority women's satisfaction depended on specific physician-expressed attitudes and associated behaviors rather than the gender of the providers.

## Physicians' Behaviors

The negative and positive interactions with physicians of different specialties, generally surgeons, radiation oncologists, and medical oncologists can be categorized into the following domains: (1) interpersonal behaviors (2) communications with partners and (3) medical expertise and decision-making.

### Interpersonal Behaviors

Physician behaviors or manners that were described as positive by women were a combination of verbal and non-verbal behaviors that led to a feeling of having rapport and established trust in the provider. Among the positive behaviors that women mentioned were making eye contact, being reassuring and compassionate towards the patient through body language, such as leaning towards the patient or reassuring the patient through physical contact. Strong agreement existed among interviewed women on the importance of good communication style:

> I like people who are trying to make some kind of connection with me, and when you translate that into the medical field, I mean you can't make a lot of connection. They're doctors. They're running fifty people through an hour. They don't have a lot of time. I like it when they make an effort to pretend they have time. You know, like I know they're still going to leave in ten minutes but they sit down and give you their full attention. And that starts for me with introducing themselves as if I were as equal a person as they are. I'm a patient and they're the doctor, but we're still human beings, and I want to be treated like a real person, not just like a patient who is a piece of meat to them. And the handshake is a connection of people. . . . Again, if they're Dr. X, I want my last name used. I'm perfectly happy for everybody to be first names. . . . But I don't want them to be a doctor and me to be a [first name].

The positive physician behaviors women commented upon were consideration, expressions of respect, seeking a connection with and showing an interest in the patient, and perceiving the patient as an equal.

Further, agreement existed on negative physician behaviors, which consisted of arrogance, challenges in communication, being dismissive, making disparaging remarks, yelling or expressing in other ways that the patient was upsetting the physician. Other negative behaviors in-

cluded keeping a patient waiting extensive amounts of time, not being
attentive, and lack of interest in the patient.

### Communications with Partners

As discussed elsewhere (Boehmer & Case, 2004), not all sexual minority women disclosed their sexual orientation to physicians, while receiving breast cancer care. For the 72% of women who disclosed their
sexual orientation (Boehmer & Case, 2004), it was important that the
physician respected them and their partner, if they chose to include their
partner in their medical appointments. One woman described meeting
her physician for the first time with her partner:

> You know, this was the first time we met. We were very up front
> [about being lesbians], and she didn't bat an eye. And she included
> [partner] in everything, talked to both of us when she was talking—
> you know, made eye contact with both of us, and I think was very
> cognizant of the fact that I was sort of in shock. And so she was
> making sure that [partner] understood what she was saying, be-
> cause it was just going in one ear and out the other, and I was just
> sitting there.

With simple changes in stance and behavior, physicians can improve
the quality of communication and care for sexual minority patients. One
area of tension is over the acceptance of same-sex partners. Most respondents reported positive interactions between partners and health
providers. One said,

> ". . . they always accepted (partner) as my spouse. [Q: Is she your
> health proxy?] Yes. Yes. And she can call my doctor, and my doc-
> tor will talk to her about what's going on."

Later, the same patient said of her treatment team

> "And my GP and my surgeon, everybody knows. I mean, every-
> body knows that [partner] is basically my mind, because usually if
> I'm in that circumstance I can't think to ask a question or what-
> ever. But they were always very good to her."

In contrast, some participants reported a more negative experience,
ranging from the subtle to the overt. One reported a difference in body
language:

"... if Dr. [Y] would hug me, she wouldn't hug her. ... if it was really emotional or upsetting, like, you have to get a mastectomy, and she would hug me, she wouldn't hug [partner], you know? But I'm not saying she had to hug the partner. ... But, ... it was distance. I don't know. It was just–it was a little–I don't know. You wouldn't necessarily hug the partner, you know. But I felt like it was a little awkward for them, just a little feeling that, like, they weren't used to having the lesbian come in the room, or they weren't comfortable with the lesbian situation–just a feeling"

Another participant reported on her physician's unwillingness to incorporate the patient's partner into care discussions, forcing the patient into translating her own care to her partner.

Dr. [X] on the other hand, had a problem and he asked her to wait outside. I said you know what? I'm not talking to you without her here. He said well, we can only talk to a spouse or you know, a family member. I said well, she's both. She's my wife and she's my family. She's my next of kin. I said you know, my mind is not clear and I'm not hearing half of the things that are being said. I want her present. I want her here. So he called her in. But when we were talking–. . . that he would address me only. He would only look at me and he would only talk to me. And then of course I would look at her and say; do you understand what he's saying? Do you have any questions? You know, and then I would turn back to him and he would–he would only address me. After the surgery and after I went back to him the first time after the surgery that he arranged for the radiation, he switched me over to a nurse practitioner. So I've never seen Dr. [X] again.

Simple changes in style and inclusion of family members in discussions (with patient consent) can result in better communication with the sexual minority patient.

## *Medical Expertise and Decision-Making*

Women commented on the advantages of a team approach and the coordination of care between different specialists. Physicians that sought the input of other specialists or did additional research were perceived as having patients' best interest at heart. Women also expressed a desire for a more comprehensive approach to cancer care and subsequently wished their treatment team included other specialists such as oncology social workers or dietitians, in addition to surgeons, radiation oncologists, and medical oncologists. One woman talked about the gaps in care:

> Well, again it's the Western medicine thing that they've pretty much just lay it on you and then leave you alone. And then leave it up to the patient to fill in the blanks so I was never talked to about diet, exercise, how to boost my immune system.

A patient-centered and participatory style was perceived as positive. Women wanted their providers to inform them about different treatments and long-term implications of breast cancer on their lives, including psychosocial and physical implications. Extensive information gave women a sense of control, while not being adequately informed about treatments and their side effects made for a negative experience. Providers who listened to patients' questions and concerns, and then answered thoroughly and in a respectful way were perceived as positive, whereas providers who were rushed, brief on details, and who discouraged questions were perceived as negative. In particular, women responded negatively to providers who presented themselves as "Gods," including being non-responsive to patients' need for information in that they discouraged patients from seeking additional information or second opinions.

> Part of my frustration with him was that he was definitely old-school. He wasn't really into you asking a lot of questions. I mean, you could ask some. But I'm a very inquisitive person. I remember going to one meeting with one other breast surgeon, and she was great. She gave me copies of my pathology report, and it was very helpful. She let me see what the pathology said. She explained it. He was not into, "this is the detail, have a copy." He was more into the kind of philosophy of "trust me I'll recommend the right thing." Which is fine, for some people. But I like having the details. I do science stuff at work.

Patients wanted guidance, explanations without intimidation, honest responses, and providers that put efforts into convincing patients of a particular treatment. Providers who voiced strong opinions about a specific treatment, while being supportive if a woman decided otherwise, were perceived as helpful.

In spite of strong agreement on what constitutes good physician behavior and care, women's expectations differed, and they made divergent choices on demanding good care. For a few women, physicians had to meet only minimal expectations to be described as good providers. In one case the absence of hostility in the patient-physician interaction was enough.

> I feel like they've all been really great actually, which again surprised me–I wasn't expecting that. . . . I feel like I used to–from the radical feminist perspective I think I expect hostility. I mean I encountered some of it in the past certainly, and I think I tend to expect it a little. I do not feel like that's been reflected in most of my medical experiences around breast cancer.

It was possible for physicians to meet these expectations and have women report their experiences as positive, because they expected being treated poorly:

> Well, I mean clearly things that I got from the support group, from friends, from community, those are needs, you know, that would be, you know, good if the doctors were very aware of: the need for including sensitivity about sexual orientation, about if anyone's overweight, you know, how that feels, to bring up body image stuff about what's going to happen, to really, really give you a lot of preparation about what's going to happen, you know, what some people's experience is like, to spend a lot of time and explain things. You know, give you a lot of hope as far as that it's temporary, and it's going to pass, and you're going to have your life back, and it will feel normal one day, you know? I think all those things would be great to hear from doctors as well, you know. And I may have even heard some of those things. But my experience wasn't negative, . . .

Other women took a different approach, and the physicians they encountered had to work harder for the patient to be satisfied:

> I feel like I'm paying them, you know? Like they're doing a job for me, and it's their job to help me, and I've seen doctors who–like that guy at [Medical Center X] who don't understand that. They don't understand that they're in a service field. (Laughter.) They think that we're there to serve them as patients, or as–you know, test cases.

While the group of women that had minimal expectations of physicians was a minority among the interviewed women, the range of what physicians had to do to be rated as a satisfying provider was an important distinction.

## DISCUSSION

In this study, we asked a community sample of 39 sexual minorities with breast cancer about their experiences with breast cancer providers. The majority of the women described increased comfort with and having a preference for female providers, confirming earlier studies that assessed lesbian patients' preferences (Geddes, 1994; Lucas, 1992). However, previous studies assessed sexual minority patients' preferences in the context of regular care or hypothetically (Geddes, 1994; Lucas, 1992), whereas our study focused on an acute and life-threatening illness. Given the fear, uncertainties, and urgency women associated with breast cancer, most did not proactively seek treatment specifically by female providers, but rather stated this preference in hindsight. Moreover, our findings indicate that participants reported on the importance of a particular communication style and certain attitudes and behaviors of providers, regardless whether the provider was male or female.

So far, evidence linking physician gender to patient satisfaction is inconsistent. Our finding of physician gender being of lesser importance compared to other physician characteristics, is consistent with earlier research of women in general that indicated being treated by female obstetricians or gynecologists is not of primary importance (Howell et al., 2002; Plunkett et al., 2002). Similarly, a questionnaire study indicated that the majority, two-thirds, had no preference for a male or female breast surgeon (Reid, 1998).

Most of the attributes that were linked by this study's sample of sexual minorities to satisfying breast cancer care confirm the results of earlier studies with patients whose sexual orientation was unidentified. Studies indicated patients' dissatisfaction with a paternalistic provider style (Allen et al., 2001; Phillips, 1996; Roter et al., 1997). Cancer patients' desire for information had been noted previously (Allen et al., 2001; Arora et al., 2002; Blanchard et al., 1988; Ong et al., 1995). Physicians' ability to listen, to communicate honestly and in a caring way, to display an interest in their patients as persons had been reported as important in an earlier breast cancer study (Harris & Templeton, 2001).

However, some of the women in our study were satisfied with providers who met minimal communication and interpersonal behavior standards, reasoning that these physicians exceeded their expectations. This suggests that sexual minority women's problems in accessing care (Institute of Medicine Committee on Lesbian Health Research Priorities, 1999) has an impact on their rating of physician behavior. We hope that future research will explore this further by using quantitative measures of patients' values and ratings of their physicians, relating these to past health care experiences and access to care.

Our hypothesis that participants would report experience with provider-patient interaction unique to sexual minority women was confirmed. Themes emerged in participants' narratives of physician experiences that went beyond the findings of studies with patients who were either heterosexual or were not identified by sexual orientation. These themes were sexual minority women's desire for a more comprehensive approach to cancer care and the need for providers' respect towards patients' sexual minority identity and their female partners. Existing studies of patients with unidentified sexual orientation indicated patients' dissatisfaction with a paternalistic provider style (Allen et al., 2001; Phillips, 1996; Roter et al., 1997). We hope that future research studies will compare sexual minorities' reactions to paternalistic provider encounters with heterosexual women's responses.

We conducted this study to investigate sexual minorities' breast cancer care–a population that is often deemed "invisible" and mostly understudied. In spite of efforts to recruit a diverse sample, an important limitation of this study is the under-representation of African American and Latina women. Our eligibility criterion of sufficient fluency in English may have compounded this problem. The mean years since diagnosis with breast cancer was 5.5 years and thus, participants' reports had the potential for recall bias. The peer-to-peer referral may have introduced bias by including and over-representing participants with similar views. While the study is limited by these biases and the findings are not generalizable to the entire population of sexual minority breast cancer patients, it is an important step toward understanding this population's preferences and particularly informative for breast cancer care providers.

Our finding that satisfaction with providers was attributed to specific traits rather than gender has important implications for provider behavior. These findings suggest that physicians of either gender can improve quality of breast cancer care for sexual minority women. While we have focused in this paper on breast cancer care providers–that is, surgeons and oncologists–the results should be informative for other health care providers who care for sexual minorities.

Physicians and providers who wish to improve their care of sexual minority patients can turn to a number of published resources that discuss the treatment of sexual minority patients and provide recommendations (Drescher, 2002; Potter, 2002; Robertson, 2005). Professional organizations such as the Gay and Lesbian Medical Association provide guidelines on the treatment of sexual minority patients (Gay and Lesbian Medical Association) and the Mautner Project has developed a video-based training program for clinicians to create awareness about lesbians' health care needs ("Removing the barriers"; Scout et al., 2001).

## REFERENCES

Allen, S. M., Petrisek, A. C., & Laliberte, L. L. (2001). Problems in doctor-patient communication: The case of younger women with breast cancer. *Critical Public Health, 11*(1), 39-58.

Arora, N. K. (2003). Interacting with cancer patients: The significance of physicians' communication behavior. *Social Science & Medicine, 57*(5), 791-806.

Arora, N. K., Johnson, P., Gustafson, D. H., McTavish, F., Hawkins, R. P., & Pingree, S. (2002). Barriers to information access, perceived health competence, and psychosocial health outcomes: Test of a mediation model in a breast cancer sample. *Patient Education and Counseling, 47*(1), 37-46.

Baile, W. F., & Aaron, J. (2005). Patient-physician communication in oncology: Past, present, and future. *Current Opinion in Oncology, 17*(4), 331-335.

Beck, R., Daughtridge, R., & Sloane, P. (2002). Physician-patient communication in the primary care office: A systematic review. *J Am Board Fam Pract, 15*(1), 25-38.

Bertakis, K. D. (1977). The communication of information from physician to patient: A method for increasing patient retention and satisfaction. *Journal of Family Practice, 5*(2), 217-22.

Bertakis, K. D., Franks, P., & Azari, R. (2003). Effects of physician gender on patient satisfaction. *Journal of the American Medical Womens Association, 58*(2), 69-75.

Bertakis, K. D., Roter, D., & Putnam, S. M. (1991). The relationship of physician medical interview style to patient satisfaction. *Journal of Family Practice, 32*(2), 175-181.

Biernacki, P., & Waldorf, D. (1981). Snowball sampling: Problems and techniques of chain referral sampling. *Sociological Methods Research, 10*(2), 141-163.

Blanchard, C. G., Labrecque, M. S., Ruckdeschel, J. C., & Blanchard, E. B. (1988). Information and decision-making preferences of hospitalized adult cancer patients. *Social Science & Medicine, 27*(11), 1139-1145.

Boehmer, U., & Case, P. (2004). Physicians don't ask, some patients tell: Disclosure of sexual orientation among women with breast cancer. *Cancer, 101*(8), 1882-1889.

Bonvicini, K. A., & Perlin, M. J. (2003). The same but different: Clinician-patient communication with gay and lesbian patients. *Patient Education & Counseling, 51*(2), 115-22.

Cochran, S. D., & Mays, V. M. (1988). Disclosure of sexual preference to physicians by black lesbian and bisexual women. *Western Journal of Medicine, 149*(5, November), 616-619.

Derose, K. P., Hays, R. D., McCaffrey, D. F., & Baker, D. W. (2001). Does physician gender affect satisfaction of men and women visiting the emergency department? *Journal of General Internal Medicine, 16*(4), 218-226.

Drescher, J. (2002). Ethical issues in treating gay and lesbian patients. *Psychiatric Clinics of North America, 25*(3), 605-621.

Elstad, J. I. (1994). Women's priorities regarding physician behavior and their preference for a female physician. *Women & Health, 21*(4), 1-19.

Fallowfield, L., & Jenkins, V. (1999). Effective communication skills are the key to good cancer care. *European Journal of Cancer, 35*(11), 1592-1597.

Gay and Lesbian Medical Association. Guidelines for care of lesbian, gay, bisexual and transgender patients. Retrieved October 27, 2005, *http://www.glma.org/pub/ GLMA_Guidelines.pdf*

Geddes, V. A. (1994). Lesbian expectations and experiences with family doctors. How much does the physician's sex matter to lesbians? *Canadian Family Physician, 40*, 908-920.

Hall, J. A., Irish, J. T., Roter, D. L., Ehrlich, C. M., & Miller, L. H. (1994). Satisfaction, gender, and communication in medical visits. *Medical Care, 32*(12), 1216-1231.

Hall, J. A., & Roter, D. L. (1998). Medical communication and gender: A summary of research. *Journal of Gender-Specific Medicine, 1*(2), 39-42.

Harris, S. R., & Templeton, E. (2001). Who's listening? Experiences of women with breast cancer in communicating with physicians. *Breast Journal, 7*(6), 444-449.

Henbest, R. J., & Stewart, M. (1990). Patient-centredness in the consultation. 2: Does it really make a difference? *Family Practice, 7*(1), 28-33.

Howell, E. A., Gardiner, B., & Concato, J. (2002). Do women prefer female obstetricians? *Obstetrics & Gynecology, 99*(6), 1031-1035.

Institute of Medicine Committee on Lesbian Health Research Priorities (Ed.). (1999). Lesbian Health. Current Assessment and Directions for the Future. Washington, DC: Institute of Medicine, Committee on Lesbian Health Research Priorities. Health Sciences Section.

Kaplan, S. H., Gandek, B., Greenfield, S., Rogers, W., & Ware, J. E. (1995). Patient and visit characteristics related to physicians' participatory decision-making style. Results from the medical outcomes study. *Medical Care, 33*(12), 1176-1187.

Klitzman, R. L., & Greenberg, J. D. (2002). Patterns of communication between gay and lesbian patients and their health care providers. *Journal of Homosexuality, 42*(4), 65-75.

Lucas, V. (1992). An investigation of the health care preferences of the lesbian population. *Health Care Women International, 13*(2), 221-228.

Matthews, A. K., Peterman, A., Delaney, P., Menard, L., & Brandenburg, D. (2002). A qualitative exploration of the experiences of lesbian and heterosexual patients with breast cancer. *Oncology Nursing Forum, 29*(10), 1455-1462.

Ong, L. M., de Haes, J. C., Hoos, A. M., & Lammes, F. B. (1995). Doctor-patient communication: A review of the literature. *Social Science & Medicine, 40*(7), 903-918.

Phillips, D. (1996). Medical professional dominance and client dissatisfaction: A study of doctor-patient interaction and reported dissatisfaction with medical care among female patients at four hospitals in Trinidad and Tobago. *Social Science & Medicine, 42*(10), 1419-25.

Plunkett, B. A., Kohli, P., & Milad, M. P. (2002). The importance of physician gender in the selection of an obstetrician or a gynecologist. *American Journal of Obstetrics & Gynecology, 186*(5), 926-928.

Potter, J. E. (2002). Do ask, do tell. *Annals of Internal Medicine, 137*(5), 341-343.

Reid, I. (1998). Patients' preference for male or female breast surgeons: Questionnaire study. *BMJ, 317*(7165), 1051.

Removing the barriers. Retrieved October 27, 2005, from *http://www.mautnerproject.org/Programs_and_Services/Healthcare_Provider_Education/*

Roberts, C. S., Cox, C. E., Reintgen, D. S., Baile, W. F., & Gibertini, M. (1994). Influence of physician communication on newly diagnosed breast patients' psychologic adjustment and decision-making. *Cancer, 74*(1 Suppl), 336-341.

Robertson, P. A. (2005). Offering high-quality ob/gyn care to lesbian patients. Retrieved September 10, 2005, from *http://www.lesbianhealthinfo.org/research/obgyn_lesbian.htm*

Roter, D. L., Hall, J. A., & Aoki, Y. (2002). Physician gender effects in medical communication: A meta-analytic review. *Jama, 288*(6), 756-764.

Roter, D. L., Stewart, M., Putnam, S. M., Lipkin, M., Jr., Stiles, W., & Inui, T. S. (1997). Communication patterns of primary care physicians. *JAMA, 277*(4), 350-356.

Scout, Bradford, J., & Fields, C. (2001). Removing the barriers: Improving practitioners' skills in providing health care to lesbians and women who partner with women. *Am J Public Health, 91*(6), 989-990.

Stein, G. L., & Bonuck, K. A. (2001). Physician-patient relationships among the lesbian and gay community. *Journal of the Gay and Lesbian Medical Association, 5*(3), 87-93.

Stewart, M., Meredith, L., Brown, J. B., & Galajda, J. (2000). The influence of older patient-physician communication on health and health-related outcomes. *Clinics in Geriatric Medicine, 16*(1), 25-36, vii-viii.

Stewart, M. A. (1995). Effective physician-patient communication and health outcomes: A review. *CMAJ Canadian Medical Association Journal, 152*(9), 1423-1433.

Strauss, A., & Corbin, J. (1990). *Basics of qualitative research: Grounded theory procedures and techniques.* Newbury Park, CA: Sage.

Watters, J. K., & Biernacki, P. (1989). Targeted sampling: Options for the study of hidden populations. *Social Problems, 36*(4), 416-430.

White, J. C., & Dull, V. T. (1998). Room for improvement: Communication between lesbians and primary care providers. *Journal of Lesbian Studies, 2*(1), 95-110.

Zachariae, R., Pedersen, C. G., Jensen, A. B., Ehrnrooth, E., Rossen, P. B., & von der Maase, H. (2003). Association of perceived physician communication style with patient satisfaction, distress, cancer-related self-efficacy, and perceived control over the disease. *British Journal of Cancer, 88*(5), 658-665.

doi:10.1300/J013v44n02_03

# Community Support, Community Values: The Experiences of Lesbians Diagnosed with Cancer

Christina Sinding, PhD
Pamela Grassau, PhD candidate
Lisa Barnoff, PhD

**SUMMARY.** The study reported in this article was initiated in response to the paucity of literature focused on Canadian lesbians with cancer. The aims of the study were broadly defined: to increase understanding of Canadian lesbians' experiences with cancer and cancer care, and to sug-

Christina Sinding is Assistant Professor, Health Studies Programme & School of Social Work, McMaster University; and Research Associate, Ontario Breast Cancer Community Research Initiative, Centre for Research in Women's Health.

Pamela Grassau is Research Associate, Ontario Breast Cancer Community Research Initiative, Centre for Research in Women's Health.

Lisa Barnoff is Assistant Professor, School of Social Work, Ryerson University.

Address correspondence to: Christina Sinding, PhD, Kenneth Taylor Hall, Room 212, McMaster University, 1280 Main Street West, Hamilton, Ontario, Canada L8S 4M4 (E-mail: sinding@mcmaster.ca).

The authors want to express their sincere appreciation to the women who agreed to be interviewed for this project, and to members of the Lesbians and Breast Cancer Project Team. This article benefited from the thorough and thoughtful attention of anonymous reviewers and the editors of *Women & Health*. *Coming Out About Lesbians and Cancer*, a community research report, is available as an HTML file and for download in PDF at www.lesbiansandcancer.com.

This research was made possible with funding from the Canadian Breast Cancer Foundation, Ontario Chapter.

[Haworth co-indexing entry note]: "Community Support, Community Values: The Experiences of Lesbians Diagnosed with Cancer." Sinding, Christina, Pamela Grassau, and Lisa Barnoff. Co-published simultaneously in *Women & Health* (The Haworth Medical Press, an imprint of The Haworth Press, Inc.) Vol. 44, No. 2, 2006, pp. 59-79; and: *Preventive Health Measures for Lesbian and Bisexual Women* (ed: Shelly Kerr, and Robin Mathy) The Haworth Medical Press, an imprint of The Haworth Press, Inc., 2006, pp. 59-79. Single or multiple copies of this article are available for a fee from The Haworth Document Delivery Service [1-800-HAWORTH, 9:00 a.m. - 5:00 p.m. (EST). E-mail address: docdelivery@haworthpress.com].

gest directions for change such that lesbians with cancer might be better supported by service providers and lesbian communities. The qualitative study, set in Ontario, Canada, employed a participatory action research model. Twenty-six lesbians were interviewed about their experiences of cancer and cancer care. This article reports research participants' narratives about lesbian community. Findings reveal the complex and sometimes contradictory ways that lesbian community unfolds in the lives of lesbians with cancer. While most participants experienced robust and competent community support, participants also reported instances of isolation and disconnection linked to fear of cancer, homophobia in the broader community, and patterns of exclusion within lesbian communities. As well, while lesbian community norms and values appeared to buffer the negative effects of treatment-related physical changes, such norms also manifested as prescriptions for lesbians with cancer. Findings affirmed the value of creating networks among lesbians with cancer within a context of increased accessibility to mainstream cancer services. doi:10.1300/J013v44n02_04 *[Article copies available for a fee from The Haworth Document Delivery Service: 1-800-HAWORTH. E-mail address: <docdelivery@haworthpress.com> Website: <http://www.HaworthPress.com> © 2006 by The Haworth Press, Inc. All rights reserved.]*

**KEYWORDS.** Lesbians, lesbian community, cancer, social support, community values

## INTRODUCTION

Over the course of the lesbian and gay liberation movement, women who had been profoundly isolated from traditional sources of social support (families, friends, faith and cultural communities) "forged communities in which they could find acceptance, understanding, and a sense of belonging" (Harper & Schneider, 2003, p. 243). Like other minorities, lesbians have had to create institutions, organizations, and rituals to serve as "social, political and psychological buffers to the hostility of the dominant culture" (Appleby & Anastas, 1998, p. 81).

Theorists often emphasize the role of lesbian and gay communities in providing a context for the emergence of social support and resources for individuals (Heaphy, Yip, & Thompson, 2004). Yet the extent to which lesbian communities actually represent alternative forms of social support are topics of debate. Some researchers (Krieger, 1982; Pisarski & Gallois, 1996) caution against overstating the extent to which lesbians are, or perceive themselves to be, supported by other lesbians. In their study in Brisbane, Australia, Pisarski and Gallois (1996) found that lesbian 'community' actually operated as a series of independent subgroups rather than a united entity. Small networks only met the needs of members for short periods of time; and, some lesbians remained isolated, in particular older lesbians. Sources of support vary according to place of residence, with urban dwellers much more likely to have access to support systems in non-heterosexual communities (Heaphy et al., 2004). Appleby and Anastas (1998) argue that racism within the lesbian community has meant that lesbians of colour do not receive the same social supports as do White lesbians. As well, Nystrom and Jones (2003) comment that, despite rhetoric and theory to the contrary, communities with limited resources often cannot meet members' needs.

Lemon and Patton (1997) note that shared values and norms are a central feature of lesbian community. While values and norms are hardly unitary among lesbians, the concept of a loosely defined 'lesbian culture' can be made workable with reference to the meeting spaces and events of community (bars, bookstores, women's rallies, and women's events) as it is in these settings that values and norms are diffused (Lemon & Patton, 1997). Lesbian culture provides an important alternative to dominant discourses about women and specifically about lesbians. At the same time, lesbian community norms and values are not always experienced as affirming; indeed, they can imply "covert management of lesbian identity by the lesbian subculture" (Lemon & Patton, 1997, 118). Extending this analysis, Dean (2005) discusses ways lesbian and gay activists, privileging visibility as central to lesbian identity, have unwittingly defined boundaries around 'what a lesbian looks like'–boundaries that exclude many lesbians. Lesbians of colour have argued that 'lesbian culture' is premised on dominant White, middle class ideals (Appleby & Anastas, 1998; Hunter, Shannon, Knox, & Martin, 1998). Given the diversity that exists among lesbians (by race, class, age, ability and place of residence) it is perhaps not surprising that ". . . there are often conflicts between the varied segments of the community" (Hunter et al., 1998, p. 46).

The current paper reports results from a qualitative study with lesbians living in Ontario, Canada who were diagnosed with breast or gynaecological cancer. To date not a single study focusing on Canadian lesbians with cancer has appeared in the literature, a gap our study intended to address. The aims of the study were broadly defined: to increase understanding of Canadian lesbians' experiences with cancer and cancer care, and to suggest directions for change such that lesbians with cancer might be better supported by service providers and lesbian communities.

Working from a subset of data from the study, this paper examines research participants' ideas about how lesbian community shaped their experiences of cancer. Participants' experiences with formal cancer care and support systems are discussed elsewhere (Barnoff, Sinding, & Grassau, in press; Sinding, Barnoff, & Grassau, 2004).

## *METHODS*

The study followed a Participatory Action Research (PAR) model. Participatory research is "systematic inquiry, with the collaboration of those affected by the issue being studied, for the purposes of education and taking action or affecting social change" (Green et al., 1995). In this model, researchers are positioned not as "separate, neutral academics theorizing about others," but rather as "co-researchers or collaborators with people working towards social equality" (Gatenby & Humphries, 2000 p. 90). The study was undertaken by a Project Team comprised of lesbians directly affected by cancer, staff and volunteers at agencies in the cancer, queer and women's health communities, and researchers. Approval for the study protocol was obtained from the Ethics Review Board at Sunnybrook and Women's College Health Sciences Centre in Toronto, Ontario.

### *Target Population, Recruitment, and Eligibility Criteria*

Lesbians living in the province of Ontario, Canada who had been diagnosed with breast cancer or gynaecological cancer at any time in the past and had been treated in Canada were eligible to participate in the study. In promotional material we defined lesbians as women whose "primary emotional and sexual relationships are with women." While the initial target population was lesbians with breast cancer, the Project Team speculated that lesbians with gynecological cancers might face very similar issues. For this reason and also to increase the number of potential study participants, lesbians with either breast or gynecological cancer were targeted for the study.

The Project Team was aware that most research in the lesbian and gay community has relied on samples "largely composed of white, middle-class, educated people with average or above average incomes living in urban areas, frequenting gay bars and identifying themselves as gay or lesbian" (Ryan, Brotman, & Rowe, 2000). We chose therefore to set explicit diversity objectives. We specified a goal of achieving diversity in the sample by race, income, education, age, ability, geographic location, identity, family status, time since diagnosis, cancer site and cancer status, and set a target for each diversity category. For example, we sought to achieve a sample in which at least one third of participants were lesbians of colour. As each participant was accrued we indicated on a chart the diversity characteristics she brought to the study; in many instances, of course, participants fit in more than one diversity category. We were aware that with a small sample it was unlikely that we would achieve the target in every diversity category; however, we deliberately set our standards high as a way of ensuring we made a serious concerted effort in relation to each one.

Our promotional material indicated intent to reflect diversity among lesbians: we wrote that we planned to interview "lesbians of colour as well as white lesbians, older and younger lesbians, lesbians with disabilities and able-bodied lesbians, lesbians living in large and small communities as well as rural areas of the province." We developed additional, community-specific promotional material to highlight the Team's particular interest in understanding the cancer and cancer care experiences of lesbians with disabilities and lesbians of colour. We also involved members of these communities in paid work related to promotion and recruitment. For instance, a lesbian living with a disability who was part of the Project Team contacted agencies serving people with disabilities to explain the study and to encourage agency staff to make their clients aware of the study.[1] We met with anti-poverty advocates to solicit ideas about reaching lesbians with cancer living in poverty and organized a teleconference with health professionals across the province to understand how best to reach lesbians with cancer living at a distance from urban centres. Further details about our efforts to achieve a diverse study sample can be found in (Sinding, Barnoff, Grassau, Odette, & McGillicuddy, submitted 2005).

The study was promoted across Ontario by staff and members of the Project Team (and, eventually, by research participants themselves). E-mail notices were circulated to service and advocacy agencies in the women's health, feminist, queer and cancer communities, and through the Project Team's personal and professional networks. Posters advertising the study were mailed to agencies listed in a province-wide directory of lesbian and gay resources.

Potential participants who contacted project staff had a chance to discuss the study on the phone or by email, and were then mailed a letter explaining the study in detail and requesting additional information (information that allowed us to track progress toward the diversity goals described above); this information was either mailed back or gathered in a follow-up phone call. In phone conversations potential participants had the opportunity to have their questions about the study answered, and to indicate a convenient time and place for the interview. All of the women who contacted the project were eligible to participate, and all confirmed in writing their voluntary, informed consent to participate.

## *Data Collection*

Interview topics focused on participants' experiences of treatment, cancer care, and support, and their feelings and ideas about any changes in body, sexuality, identity and relationships. Interviews (one and a half hours in length on average) were tape recorded and transcribed. Face-to-face interviews (n = 17) were conducted at times and in locations comfortable and convenient for participants, either in their homes or at our research offices. Telephone interviews (n = 9) were conducted at a time convenient to participants when they were in settings where conversation was comfortable and confidential. A $30 honourarium was provided for participating and completing the interview.

Twenty-six lesbians diagnosed with cancer (twenty-two with breast cancer, three with gynecological cancer, one with both) were interviewed over a six month period beginning in January 2003. Names associated with the quotes were chosen by participants.

## *Data Analysis*

Once five interviews had been completed, each member of the Project Team reviewed three transcripts, and met to discuss emergent themes. Drawing from detailed minutes taken at that meeting as well as the research team's review and discussion of an additional seven transcripts, a coding framework was developed. Transcripts were coded using the qualitative software program NVivo (Bazeley & Richards, 2000). The research team discussed the coding framework at length, and independently coded three transcripts to ensure reliability. Further interviews were coded as they were completed and new codes were added as necessary.

A central aim of this study was to understand more fully lesbians' cancer experiences. In relation to this aim, participants' reports of how their partners and friends and the broader lesbian community responded (or failed to respond) to their diagnoses emerged as an important theme. In exploring this theme, we employed the key grounded theory method of attending to the conditions under which phenomena arose and the consequences associated with a phenomenon (Strauss & Corbin, 1990). Specifically we examined why participants believed they were supported (or not supported) and we examined the effect that support (or lack of it) had on the participant.

Early in the analysis the Team also focused on instances in which participants made comments that linked 'being a lesbian' with the cancer experience. Participants' statements about what cancer is or should be like for lesbians–including how lesbians (should) react to cancer, and how lesbians (should) support lesbians who are ill–were discussed. While we did not initially perceive these statements as directly relevant to the idea of 'community,' analytic memos (Strauss & Corbin, 1990) focused on these findings eventually led us to conceptualize them as reflections of community norms and values.

These two sub-sets of the overall data–one centred on perceptions of support in community, and the other on community norms and values–form the basis for this paper. While we did not intend in our analysis to create typologies or formal theory, we did, as noted, employ key grounded theory methods (Strauss & Corbin, 1994; Charmaz, 2000), including constant comparison within and between accounts. In particular, both to adhere to principles of qualitative analysis (Seale, 1999) and to minimize the risk of stereotyping lesbians, negative cases (instances in which participants' experiences or commentary departed from or challenged an emerging theme) were examined and reported.

## FINDINGS

Table 1 displays the demographic characteristics of the 26 study participants.

### Support in Lesbian Community

In considering participants' perceptions of community support, we first examined the theme of a 'lesbian advantage' in support. We then considered a counter theme: isolation and disconnection from other lesbians. In the section that follows, we explored participants' ideas about barriers to support.

TABLE 1. Demographic characteristics of research participants

| | |
|---|---|
| *Age* | Average age 50 years; range = 36-72 years |
| *Time since diagnosis* | Three years or more: 13; less than three years: 13 |
| *Place of birth* | Canada: 20; United States: 2; England: 1; The Philippines: 1; Jamaica: 1; Hong Kong: 1 |
| *First language* | English: 24; Cree: 1; Dutch: 1 |
| *Race/ethnicity (self-defined)[a]* | Caucasian/White : 7; British: 6; Canadian: 2; Jewish: 2; Indigenous/Native 2; Metis-Ukrainian 1; Euro Canadian 1; Polish Canadian: 1; Italian : 1; Asian: 1 |
| *Total annual household income (Canadian dollars)* | $100,000+ – 6     $70-79,000 – 2     $40-49,000 – 1     Less than $20,000 – 1[b] $90-99,000 – 1     $60-69,000 – 3     $30-39,000 – 4 $80-89,000 – 1     $50-59,000 – 4     $20-29,000 – 2 |
| *Education* | University degree: 19; College diploma: 6; Secondary school diploma: 1 |
| *Disability/health problems aside from cancer* | One woman is hearing impaired; one has heart problems and arthritis and is a psychiatric survivor; one has experienced depression and has fibromyalgia; one has endometriosis. |
| *Urban/rural (at time of treatment)* | Urban: 20; semi-urban: 2; rural: 4. |
| *Family status (at diagnosis)* | Partnered: 17; Single: 9. Adult children: 5; young children: 1; trying to have children: 2. |
| *Identity* | Lesbian: 22; Gay: 2; Dyke: 1; Bisexual: 1. |
| *Family doctor knew identity* | Yes: 23; No: 2; not sure: 1. |

[a] One woman said the question was impossible to answer as her ethnicity was "too mixed"; one did not respond.
[b] Actual income ~ $8000; one woman did not respond.

## *'The Lesbian Advantage' in Support*

The majority of participants in this study reported receiving substantial and much valued support from lesbian partners and friends. Several, in fact, made the claim that lesbians are 'better off' than heterosexual women in terms of support and care. This perception of relative advantage had two main components: the perception that women are especially empathic and the assessment that support provided by lesbians is especially competent and well-organized.

Some of the women interviewed spoke of feeling exceptionally well-understood by lesbian partners and friends. Rosalie speculated that her partner's gender may be a factor in how present and connected emotionally she was able to be:

> My partner has a woman's point of view, a woman's experience that . . . you can just be quiet together and not have to fix anything . . . I don't know if it's because she's a woman or not, but my partner is very able to talk about her feelings and my feelings.

Reflecting on the care her partner and friends offered, Geri said: "I think that [my partner] understood how I felt about certain things because she's a woman. . . . I just think that women are softer and more caring, oh that's a bad thing to say, but I do believe it!" Rosalie further suggested that the shared experience of a woman's body contributes to lesbian partners' capacities for empathy:

> My partner has ovaries. My partner has a uterus. My partner could be in my position. My partner knows what it's like to live in our world and have a uterus and ovaries. My partner knows that it can be difficult to talk about in general society. My partner knows what a check-up means, and submitting to all that poking.

Other participants described their lesbian friends as especially competent, and claimed they offered exceptionally well-organized care. Sherry, for instance, said:

> I could have asked for anything but I didn't have to, I mean, they said, "we're here, what do you need?" You know, they're dykes . . . Do you need food, do you need a drive . . . you need a phone call? They just like, started taking care of stuff, you know what I mean?

In Sherry's assessment, 'taking care of things' and 'being a dyke' are virtually synonymous. In keeping with this idea, several participants noted that the process of figuring out how to provide care for gay male friends with AIDS has meant that lesbians have a store of knowledge about how to make care teams and networks successful. Mary Lou, for instance, described "this incredible support network that worked liked a charm," that allowed her to "just be sick and not worry about things." As Mary Lou saw it, it was the skills one particular woman brought, along with a community experience of caring for men with AIDS, that lent the support network such a high degree of organization and effectiveness. Lillian suggested, further, that connections among lesbians are linked to resources:

> The community is three inches by five, so if you need X, that might not be in your immediate circle but somebody you know slept with somebody who knows somebody who can get X, you know what I mean. . . . it's sort of concentric circles or what I like to refer to as the 'great lesbian chart.'

The 'great lesbian chart' worked well for several of the women we interviewed. Paula K., for instance, spoke about how lesbians she did not know well at all before her diagnosis started bringing her meals when she became ill. Where community is strong, one lesbian's diagnosis with cancer can generate a community response, drawing lesbians beyond her immediate circle into a network of support (Sinding, 1999).

## *Isolation and Disconnection*

While support from the lesbian community was most often perceived as abundant and effective, the majority of lesbians who took part in this research also experienced at least some instances of feeling and being isolated and disconnected from their partners, and from the broader lesbian community.

Some research participants had experiences that ran directly counter to the ideals discussed above, of lesbians providing superior emotional support and communicating especially well:

> [The woman I was with at the time] was wonderful in dealing with the logistics, she really was. I mean she's a nurse, she had me well looked after. But she couldn't cope with my emotional reactions. She didn't know what to do. [Liz]

> [My partner and I] didn't hardly communicate, or we didn't talk about the cancer hardly at all . . . so it was really hard. [Theresa]

> Even in the lesbian community, lesbians have a difficult time with [cancer], you know, I had a couple of friends that I don't talk to anymore–'you can come with us, you can do whatever but don't talk about the cancer.' [Glenda]

For these research participants, shared identity did not appear to facilitate empathy from partners. Further, the specific shared experience of a woman's body did not always ease isolation or distress; in fact, it sometimes seemed to exacerbate it. Kate noted that when two women are being sexual after one has had a woman's cancer, it is difficult to avoid awareness of the cancer. The mirror of the other body shows a change, an absence, a loss: "the fact that my body and her body are different in that way is always present in that relationship." As well, as Sarah pointed out, lesbians know what it is like to touch another woman's body sexually, so when a lesbian loses a breast, she knows what her sexual partner misses in a very personal, physical way. The sameness of bodies in a lesbian relationship, while on the one hand a source of understanding, may make the consequences of treatment for a woman's cancer especially complex and difficult in lesbian partnerships.

For one woman, shared identity lent challenges to support from friends as well. Theresa speaking about her friends' reactions to her diagnosis, said this:

> I think lesbians really identify with their breasts, you know, as a sexual thing. . . . And then it becomes like 'wow, what if I lost mine . . . how horrible would that be, you know? Who'd want to touch me?'

Teresa was surprised to find that she was in some ways better supported by her gay male friends than her lesbian friends. The gay men in her life wanted to know the details about what it was like for her on a daily basis to live with cancer. Talking about her lesbian friends, Theresa said, "I mean they all came, they were all very good, they came in shifts to the hospital and stuff, right? But . . . I think it was very hard on them."

Finally, support at a community level was not always perceived to be competent or well organized. Describing how other lesbians responded to her cancer diagnosis, Lillian said this:

> Telling other lesbians that you have cancer is a very brave act. It's funny, you could probably tell them that you are HIV positive, and you'd get more . . . like people wouldn't be as creepy, because there's been enough in the community about being supportive, and it's not so bad and everything. But cancer scares the shit out of people, and they don't know what to do with you. It's really weird. And that part I didn't expect.

Lillian suggests that lesbian communities are not yet fully engaged with responding to cancer. As difficult as it is to hear about an HIV diagnosis, she says, it is familiar; lesbians have some collective sense of competence about providing support for men and women with HIV. As Lillian perceives it, lesbian community competence is not yet established in relation to cancer. For Marcia, it was the comparison of her own experience to what she saw happen for men with AIDS that revealed lesbian support and organizing in relation to cancer lacking:

> I did not feel that I had a lot of support from the lesbian community. . . . I think that the lesbian community has to wrestle with body stuff, aging stuff . . . you know, how do we care for each other, rather than how do we care for the boys. I think we did a terrific job in terms of the HIV/AIDS epidemic, but . . .

Marcia went on to describe ways that lesbians could begin to create support for lesbians with cancer within existing services. Along with other participants, she highlighted the importance of formal lesbian-positive cancer services where informal networks are not strong and in situations where care is needed over long periods of time, a point to which we return.

### Barriers to Support

Over the course of interviews, some participants reflected on the barriers to community support for lesbians with cancer. Fear was the key theme; also relevant was homophobia and other patterns of privilege and oppression operating in the larger society.

Fear of cancer affects lesbian communities, as Sarah pointed out:

> There's five of us [lesbians] in [city] with breast cancer and two have died in the last 12 months, so people are scared. Yeah, what makes it more scary is the fact that the women who died were the leaders of the community, they were the ones who coordinated the dances, coffee houses and everything like that so they were very visible so it scares women.

These fears directly affected the support received by participants. Sarah kept her cancer diagnosis hidden because of her awareness of this fear, particularly because she felt it would compromise potential relationships. Yet as she attempted to protect the possibility of relationship for herself by not revealing her diagnosis, Sarah was unable to draw on community support for her experience with cancer. Worry about how a potential partner will react to learning about cancer is something both lesbians and heterosexual women with cancer experience. Yet lesbians' worries about forming partnerships occur in a context in which dating can be a challenge, as homophobia and heterosexism limit lesbians' capacities to be visible to each other and within the wider society.

In addition, some participants argued that the fear lesbians have about cancer means that each lesbian diagnosed became a symbol for all lesbians of the threat of the disease. This could also be a barrier to support, as Marcia explains: "I did feel invisible as a cancer survivor, in the lesbian community . . . [I] felt like I represented the fear of all lesbians, of getting breast cancer."

The isolation research participants experienced was also linked to homophobia in the broader community. Participants living outside urban centres pointed out that the 'great lesbian chart' does not work well—or at all—for them. Laura explained that homophobia in small and rural communities "leads you not to have friends as much, it leads you not to have support." Marcia echoed this point:

> I'm in [county] and . . . all gays and lesbians are mostly invisible up here. There are no gay and lesbian resources up here. And so . . . well, that simply makes me sad in terms of, you know, good grief, it's 2003 and there are still parts of Ontario that are completely in the closet.

Finally, one participant, Glenda, spoke about being excluded from cancer support centres and services because they assumed and required a level of financial resources that she, living on social assistance, does not have. It was not only the failure of formal service providers to provide the costs of transportation or the fees associated with self-care initiatives that proved a barrier, however; it was also other women with cancer taking their resources for granted:

> Having the doctor say, you know, "you've got that big C" that's bad enough and then sitting in these groups and these women are talking about going on these retreats and they're talking about these juicers and they're talking about all this stuff . . . These women are talking about juicers and I'm sitting there thinking, 'juicers? Like . . . I don't [even] have juice . . .'

Axtell (1999) argues that broad social stratifications along the lines of class, race and ability operate in lesbian communities. Glenda's comments were not made specifically in relation to other lesbians with cancer, but her comments pointed to the ways patterns of privilege and disadvantage among women may compromise support.

## Lesbian 'Culture,' Values, and Norms: Effects on Lesbians with Cancer

In examining participants' perceptions of how lesbian community values and norms informed their experiences, we again considered 'the lesbian advantage,' the ways that lesbian community values provided a positive resource to lesbians diagnosed with cancer. We then explored ways that community values were irrelevant, not enacted, or perceived as problematic.

*The Lesbian Advantage:*
*Community Values as a Positive Resource*

Many women diagnosed with cancer cut their hair short before chemotherapy. Short hair may, however, have different meanings for lesbians than it does for heterosexual women. Dean (2005) suggests that short hair has historically been among the signifiers of lesbian identity. For some of the lesbians who participated in this research, then, having very short hair, a shaved head or being bald was linked with a positive lesbian self-image:

> I have a wonderful butch lesbian friend who taught me how to do my hair with one of those hair-clipper things. I had never done that before in my life. [laughter] And as a [professional], I always struggled with, 'OK, so, how dykey can my hair go and still pass, still be acceptable . . .' So it was the first time I could have a legitimate absolute dyke haircut. And so for me it was liberating . . . [and] sort of in tune with, we're queer, we're here, and we're not going away! [Marcia]

Mary Lou spoke of a similar experience; after her hair grew back, she continued to shave her head. "It's given me the freedom just to go–it's given me the excuse to be able to look, well, to look butch!" Paddy said, "the cutting of my hair essentially was my way of saying to the world, 'I'm still a butch'" in the face of the threat from cancer. In these women's stories, having very short hair was a way of affirming a lesbian or a butch identity and a way of maintaining or connecting to power.

Constance spoke about another connection between hair loss and being a lesbian with cancer:

> [In the queer community] they're like, "yeah, you go girl . . ." I still have one waiter at [restaurant] who always says, "when are you going to shave your head again, I love that, you look so great." I finally told him a couple of months ago why I didn't have hair then, he went, "really, well you still look fabulous" and I thought, 'love you'. That was the kind of support we got, you know.

In queer community, Constance suggests, a bald woman is not necessarily seen as a woman with cancer. This meant that Constance was, as she says, treated "like a normal human being."

Perceived norms around the body also affected the lesbians we interviewed. Some participants believe that lesbians as a community rely less than do heterosexual women on the social symbols of womanhood, including breasts, and are thus less affected by breast loss:

> I think definitely, for lesbians–at least this is the way I feel–that it is not a priority for them to go out and get reconstructive surgery . . . I think heterosexual women have more pressures about the fact that they have to have breasts to be a woman. Whereas I didn't feel that way at all. I didn't feel any less of a woman, in any way, losing my right breast. [Jacquie]

Jacquie went on to speak about the tattoo she designed for her chest, and how other lesbians "really admired me getting the tattoo, and the strength behind it." In keeping with this analysis, Martindale (1994) suggests that lesbian feminists, particularly Audre Lorde (1992), have offered women with breast cancer the means to identify and resist the heterosexism inherent in medical discussions of breast reconstruction, and to claim visibility and pride as breastless women.

Several participants felt that lesbians struggle less with breast loss than do heterosexual women because their partners assign less value to breasts than (heterosexual) men would. Laura told a story about a young woman whose male partner left her when she had a mastectomy:

> I think a woman has more empathy towards that if it was her partner, I mean she wouldn't drop her partner because a woman doesn't have breasts . . . it's more of an emotional love than a physical fixation . . . If I had had a mastectomy or had some disfigurement of my breast, it would be more acceptable with another woman than it would be with a man.

Perceived community norms about the body, including a rejection of the idea that breasts define womanhood and sexuality, shaped these women's experiences. Participants quoted here suggest that lesbians with cancer are less negatively affected by breast loss than are heterosexual women.

## Community Norms Irrelevant, Not Enacted, or Problematic

While most participants who commented about hair loss reported feeling supported by lesbian community norms, some participants in this research found nothing good or normal or powerful at all about losing their hair. Rosalie, for instance, loved her long hair, and found it "so hard to go bald." For Teagan, losing hair during chemotherapy was part of "not feeling human." And Laura said this:

> You feel like in a way you've died and been reborn. Your hair goes right down below the skin line, it takes months for it to even come back, I'd never seen my bare head since I was a baby, and . . . Oh, it was dreadful, I hid away from people . . . . If they would have said, 'what's the worst time of your life?' I naturally would say, 'when I was on chemo.'

While community norms allowed some lesbians who took part in this research to buffer the difficult impact of hair loss, or even to find power in it, it was clear that hair loss disrupted identity and was traumatic and disempowering for others.

In a few instances, perceived norms about the body were not enacted: breast loss did affect research participants' partners and potential partners in negative ways. One participant who spoke about this issue referred to the strength she initially drew from "the lesbian belief" that changes to her appearance would not affect her desirability or lovability:

> [At the time of my surgery] I had that lesbian belief in my head, it doesn't matter what I look like, lesbians are going to love me anyway. So I had that in my head, no problem, no matter what I look like, I'm strong and this isn't going to bother me. [Glenda]

It was especially hard, then, to find that this belief–this community value–was not always enacted, and that changes to her breast did matter: "Some women don't even want to look at that breast, some women don't even want to touch that breast, some women you never hear from again."

In at least one case, a participant perceived lesbian community values about the body as actively problematic. Lillian, considering breast reconstruction, had this experience:

I read some stuff, little bits and pieces about lesbian breast cancer survivors . . . There's a lot of it about the patriarchy forcing implants upon you and you know these horrible chemical things and how awful it was. And [lesbians saying] 'I was proud to not have boobs'. It was like that, sort of strange judgmental bit about, you know, somebody wants to be femmy, 'oh, well, they're just passing' . . .

*Interviewer: So, how did that make you feel?*

Oh, the usual, you know, you're not part of the group, you're being culled from the herd.

In Lillian's analysis, breast reconstruction had been constituted in lesbian community as a form of 'passing,' a bid for respectability in relation to dominant (heterosexual) values. As Dean points out, lesbian community process of identity management have important, and sometimes negative, consequences:

An erasure or dismissal causes some lesbians to struggle precisely with this question of whether we qualify as 'real' lesbians or not, putting our sense of identity in crisis and sometimes resulting in our ostracism from lesbian community. (Dean, 2005, p. 97)

## *DISCUSSION*

Participants in this study were not representative of lesbians with cancer; the findings are, thus, not generalizable. While we do not have baseline data on Canadian lesbians for comparison, it is reasonable to assume that this particular sample was better educated and wealthier than the general population of lesbians. Despite considerable effort, the sample was also largely white, and few lesbians with disabilities participated (for further discussion, see Sinding et al., submitted 2005). Selection bias may have resulted from how the study was promoted: the term 'lesbian,' for instance, may be less likely to draw older participants than the term 'gay woman,' and reliance on written, English-language promotional material meant that women who are unable to read, or unable to read English, did not participate. Participation bias was also a factor, as lesbians who chose to take part were likely to be those better connected to the lesbian community.

In the context of these limitations, analysis revealed considerable variation in participants' perceptions and experiences of support in lesbian community, and sometimes-contradictory affects on their well-being of lesbian community norms and values.

Shared identity was often a basis for empathy and connection, and a majority of participants who were part of lesbian communities felt they were supported in especially caring and effective ways. Yet shared identity was clearly not always sufficient: participants reported many instances of isolation and disconnection, and, for some, isolation from other lesbians characterized their experience. In a few instances, shared identity also proved a kind of liability for lesbians with cancer. Lesbians, witnessing 'one of our own' diagnosed with breast or gynecological cancer, may identify with her in ways that make support awkward or impossible. The diagnosis of a woman's cancer in the context of two women's bodies may also, this research suggests, complicate intimacy and sexuality.

Part of shared identity for lesbians is a history of supporting gay men with AIDS. Participants in this study suggested that the AIDS movement served as a touchstone for lesbians with cancer. The social movement that AIDS prompted was an example from which lesbians with cancer would sometimes draw in a positive way, as testament to what is possible when marginalized communities organize in response to illness. At the same time the AIDS movement served as evidence of a collective response–of empathy, resources, services and advocacy–that has yet to be mobilized for lesbians with cancer in Canada.

A key challenge to support for lesbians with cancer was fear. Research participants noted that fear about cancer–perhaps especially acute in relation to 'women's cancers'–operated at a community level, compromising support in a range of ways. Further challenges to support stemmed from homophobia in the broader community, and patterns of exclusion (along lines of income and race, for instance) that operate in lesbian communities, both of which rendered genuine community scarce. The impact of socioeconomic status on community-based support networks merits careful attention. Among participants in Aronson's (1998, p. 514) study, for instance, were women whose support networks were small and "stretched for resources of all kinds and, as a result . . . quite strained and fragile."

Lesbian community norms and values also hold contradictory possibilities. On the one hand, the challenge lesbians present to dominant notions of how women (should) look opens spaces for lesbians with cancer (Martindale, 1994), allowing for the possibility of power and pleasure in hair loss, and the potential that breast loss is experienced as less devastating than it often is for heterosexual women. Yet as participants in this research noted, alternative values did not always translate into practice. As well, lesbians' challenge to prevailing constructions of womanhood may manifest as prescriptions: at least one lesbian who chose breast reconstruction perceived judgement about 'selling out' to dominant (heterosexual) cultural norms.

Asked to consider the changes they wished to see for lesbians with cancer in Ontario, participants in this research called for the creation of "safe" spaces. Key among their recommendations were mechanisms to foster connections among lesbians diagnosed with cancer: support and wellness groups, and one-to-one telephone support and information systems. Existing literature echoes these recommendations. Fobair and colleagues (2002), for instance, note the numerous positive benefits which emerged for lesbians diagnosed with cancer as a result of being in a lesbian-only therapy group. Such opportunities are only just emerging for Canadian lesbians with cancer (but see Boehmer (2000) for an account of lesbian-specific services in the U.S., and of lesbians' activism in the U.S. cancer movement).

Findings from the current study have implications for networks of lesbians with cancer. Such networks may provide the basis for organizing and activism that leads to more abundant support for lesbians who are ill. The research reported here suggests that particular attention is merited in these efforts to countering fear of cancer in lesbian communities and to fully attending to the support needs of lesbians outside urban centres, and lesbians living in poverty. Further, networks among lesbians with cancer offer an opportunity for exploring how lesbian community values and norms shape lesbians' cancer experiences. In safe spaces, lesbians with cancer may have a chance to more fully embrace those norms and values that lend strength and courage, and to challenge and reject those that do not.

More generally, however, as sustaining and liberating as community-based care and cultural values may be in a particular health crisis for particular lesbians, this research confirms that at the current historical moment, 'community' is insufficient and sometimes problematic in relation to many lesbians' cancer-related needs and experience. As other researchers have noted (particularly in relation to lesbians of colour (Appleby & Anastas, 1998), and as is confirmed by this study, some lesbians get left out or shut out of 'community.' In order for all lesbians with cancer to receive adequate support, then, mainstream cancer services must ensure their accessibility to lesbians and lesbian families

(Sinding et al., 2004). This study thus echoes Aronson's (1998) caution that the efforts lesbians devote towards fostering community be part of a larger vision, in which care and support for people from marginalized communities is a central objective not only for those particular communities, but also for social and public policy.


## NOTE

1. Members of the Project Team took on focused recruitment with communities of which they were members not because the rest of the Team expected them to represent the entire community, but because we believed that lesbians of colour with cancer, and lesbians with disabilities with cancer, would be more likely to find the project credible because a lesbian of colour and a lesbian with a disability were active on the Team.


## REFERENCES

Appleby, G. A., & Anastas, J. W. (1998). *Not Just a Passing Phase: Social Work with Gay, Lesbian, and Bisexual People.* New York: Columbia University Press.

Aronson, J. (1998). Lesbians giving and receiving care: Stretching conceptualizations of caring and community. *Women's Studies International Forum, 21*(5), 509-519.

Axtell, S. (1999). Disability and chronic illness identity: Interviews with lesbians and bisexual women and their partners. *Journal of Gay, Lesbian and Bisexual Identity, 4*(1), 53-72.

Barnoff, L., Sinding, C., & Grassau, P. (in press). Lesbians diagnosed with cancer: Experiences of cancer support services and recommendations for change. *Journal of Gay and Lesbian Social Services, 18*(1).

Bazeley, P., & Richards, L. (2000). *NVivo Qualitative Project Book.* London: Sage Publications.

Boehmer, U. (2000). *The personal and the Political: Women's Activism in Response to the Breast Cancer and AIDS Epidemics.* Albany: State University of New York.

Charmaz, K. (2000). Grounded Theory: Objectivist and constructivist methods. In N. Denzin & Y. Lincoln (Eds.), *Handbook of Qualitative Research* (Vol. 2, pp. 509-535). Thousand Oaks, CA: Sage Publications.

Dean, A. (2005). Does a lesbian need a vagina like a fish needs a bicycle? Or would the 'real' lesbian please stand up! *Canadian Women's Studies, 24*(2/3), 93-101.

Fobair, P., Koopman, C., DiMiceli, S., O'Hanlan, K., Butler, L. D., Classen, C., et al. (2002). Psychosocial intervention for lesbians with primary breast cancer. *Psycho-oncology, 11*(5), 427-438.

Gatenby, B., & Humphries, M. (2000). Feminist participatory action research: Methodological and ethical issues. *Women's Studies International Forum, 23*(1), 89-105.

Green, L. W., George, M. A., Daniel, M., Frankish, C. J., Herbert, C. J., Bowie, W. R., et al. (1995). *Study of Participatory Research in Health Promotion/Review and Recommendations for the Development of Participatory Research in Health Pro-*

*motion in Canada.* Institute of Health Promotion Research, the University of British Columbia, and the B.C. Consortium for Health Promotion Research.

Harper, G., & Schneider, M. (2003). Oppression and discrimination among lesbian, gay, bisexual and transgendered people and communities: A challenge for community psychology. *American Journal of Community Psychology, 31*(3/4), 243-252.

Heaphy, B., Yip, A., & Thompson, D. (2004). Ageing in a non-heterosexual context. *Ageing and Society, 24*, 881-902.

Hunter, S., Shannon, C., Knox, J., & Martin, J. (1998). *Lesbian, Gay, and Bisexual Youth and Adults: Knowledge for Human Services Practice.* Thousand Oaks: Sage.

Krieger, S. (1982). Lesbian identity and community: Recent social science literature. Signs: *Jounal of Women in Culture and Society, 8*, 91-108.

Lemon, G., & Patton, W. (1997). Lavender blue: Issues in lesbian identity development with a focus on an Australian lesbian community. *Women's Studies International Forum, 20*(1), 113-127.

Lorde, A. (1992). *The Cancer Journals* (Vol. 2). San Francisco: Aunt Lute Books.

Martindale, K. (1994). Can I get a witness? My lesbian breast cancer story. *Fireweed, 42*(Winter), 9-15.

Nystrom, N., & Jones, T. (2003). Community building with aging and old lesbians. *American Jounal of Community Psychology, 31*(3/4), 293-300.

Pisarski, A., & Gallois, C. (1996). A needs analysis of Brisbane lesbians: Implications for the lesbian community. *Journal of Homosexuality, 30*(4), 79-95.

Ryan, B., Brotman, S., & Rowe, B. (2000). *Access to Care: Exploring the Health and Well-Being of Gay, Lesbian, Bisexual and Two-Spirit People in Canada.* Montreal: McGill Centre for Applied Family Studies.

Seale, C. (1999). *The Quality of Qualitative Research.* London: Sage Publications.

Sinding, C. (1999). Counting on desire: Supporting a lesbian with breast cancer. In M. Denton, M. Hadjukowski-Ahmed, M. O'Connor & I. U. Zeytinoglu (Eds.), *Women's Voices in Health Promotion* (pp. 191-203). Toronto: Canadian Scholars Press.

Sinding, C., Barnoff, L., & Grassau, P. (2004). Homophobia and heterosexism in cancer care: Lesbians' experiences. *Canadian Journal of Nursing Research, 36*(4), 170-188.

Sinding, C., Barnoff, L., Grassau, P., Odette, F., & McGillicuddy, P. (submitted 2005). The story we tell: The processes and politics of representation. In J. Gould, J. Nelson & S. Keller-Olman (Eds.), *Searching for Knowledge: Encouraging Change: Participatory Research in Cancer Contexts (working title).*

Strauss, A., & Corbin, J. (1990). *Basics of Qualitative Research: Grounded Theory Procedures and Techniques.* Newbury Park, CA: Sage.

Strauss, A., & Corbin, J. (1994). Grounded theory methodology: An overview. In N. Denzin & Y. Lincoln (Eds.), *Handbook of Qualitative Research* (pp. 273-285). Thousand Oaks, CA: Sage Publications.

doi:10.1300/J013v44n02_04

# Psychosocial Responses to Treatment for Breast Cancer Among Lesbian and Heterosexual Women

Patricia L. Arena, PhD
Charles S. Carver, PhD
Michael H. Antoni, PhD
Sharlene Weiss, PhD
Gail Ironson, MD, PhD
Ron E. Durán, PhD

**SUMMARY.** This study compared the experiences of 39 self-identified lesbians and 39 heterosexual women who had recently been treated for breast cancer. They were matched by age, stage of disease, time since diagnosis, and ethnicity. Data were collected by a questionnaire completed at home and returned by mail. Variables assessed included emotional adjustment, thought intrusion and avoidance, perceived quality of life, concerns about breast cancer, benefit finding, relationship and sex-

Patricia L. Arena, Charles S. Carver, Michael H. Antoni, Sharlene Weiss, Gail Ironson, and Ron E. Durán are affiliated with the University of Miami.

Address correspondence to: Patricia L. Arena, PhD, Cherokee Health Systems, 815 West 5th North Street, Morristown, TN 37814 (E-mail: Patricia.Arena@cherokeehealth. com).

This research was supported by funding from the National Cancer Institute (CA64710). Patricia Arena is now at Cherokee Health Systems, Morristown, TN. Ron Durán is now at Alliant International University, Alhambra, CA.

[Haworth co-indexing entry note]: "Psychosocial Responses to Treatment for Breast Cancer Among Lesbian and Heterosexual Women." Arena, Patricia L. et al. Co-published simultaneously in *Women & Health* (The Haworth Medical Press, an imprint of The Haworth Press, Inc.) Vol. 44, No. 2, 2006, pp. 81-102; and: *Preventive Health Measures for Lesbian and Bisexual Women* (ed: Shelly Kerr, and Robin Mathy) The Haworth Medical Press, an imprint of The Haworth Press, Inc., 2006, pp. 81-102. Single or multiple copies of this article are available for a fee from The Haworth Document Delivery Service [1-800-HAWORTH, 9:00 a.m. - 5:00 p.m. (EST). E-mail address: docdelivery@haworthpress.com].

Available online at http://wh.haworthpress.com
doi:10.1300/J013v44n02_05

ual disruption, psychosexual adjustment, social support, and coping. Compared to the heterosexual women, lesbians reported less thought avoidance, lower levels of sexual concern, less concern about their appearance, and less disruption in sexual activity, but also substantially lower perceptions of benefit from having had cancer. Lesbians reported less social connection to family, but no group difference emerged in connection to friends. Lesbians reported less denial coping, and more use of support from friends, more venting, and more positive reframing. Better understanding of the similarities and differences between groups will help address the relevant clinical issues appropriately, in order to optimize psychosocial adjustment to breast cancer. *doi:10.1300/J013v44n02_05 [Article copies available for a fee from The Haworth Document Delivery Service: 1-800-HAWORTH. E-mail address: <docdelivery@haworthpress.com> Website: <http://www.HaworthPress.com> © 2006 by The Haworth Press, Inc. All rights reserved.]*

**KEYWORDS.** Breast cancer, lesbian, coping, social support, psychosexual, benefit finding

Breast cancer is the most frequently diagnosed cancer and the second leading cause of death among women in the US (American Cancer Society, 2005). Currently, it is believed that most women diagnosed with early stage breast cancer return to normal levels of emotional adjustment within about a year after diagnosis (for reviews see Glanz & Lerman, 1992; Moyer & Salovey, 1996). Nevertheless, being diagnosed with breast cancer still represents a significant stressor in a woman's life. Adverse psychosocial reactions to the diagnosis and treatment of breast cancer are important in their own right, because of the suffering involved, and also because they can interfere with patient adherence to medical regimens (e.g., Williamson, 2000). Such psychosocial responses to breast cancer are the focus of this article.

The vast majority of research concerning women's reactions to breast cancer comes from studies of middle-class non-Hispanic White heterosexual women. Consequently, relatively little has been known until recently about reactions to breast cancer among women who are ethnic and sexual minorities. Research on the experience of various ethnic minorities is beginning to emerge. For example, several studies have found that African-American women tend to report less distress and concern for the future than do non-Hispanic White women, who report less distress and disruption than Hispanic women (e.g., Culver, Arena,

Antoni, & Carver, 2002; Culver, Arena, Wimberly, Antoni, & Carver, 2004; Spencer et al., 1999).

Until very recently, information regarding the psychological and emotional experiences of sexual minority women with breast cancer has been almost entirely lacking. Several studies have begun to change that picture, however. One recent qualitative study explored the experiences of lesbian and heterosexual women who had been treated for breast cancer within the preceding 5 years, using focus groups of 4-8 participants (Matthews, Peterman, Delaney, Menard, & Brandenburg, 2002). Lesbians reported greater stress from diagnosis and treatment and less satisfaction with treatment, compared to heterosexual women. In most other respects, however, the groups resembled each other to a considerable degree.

Another recent study compared psychosocial responses to breast cancer among 29 lesbian women and 246 heterosexuals (Fobair et al., 2001). In that study lesbians reported less body image concern than heterosexuals. Lesbians also reported less avoidance of thoughts about the cancer than did heterosexual women but tended to have more involuntary thought intrusions (at the .07 level). The groups did not differ in sexual functioning or reported sexual satisfaction either before or after breast cancer, and they did not differ in self-reported distress. Fobair et al. (2001) found that lesbians (more than heterosexuals) reported that their partners made them feel loved and cared for, were willing to listen, and could be counted on to help with daily tasks. Heterosexuals, on the other hand, found their partners too demanding, more than did lesbians. Heterosexual women reported relying on relatives for help and support more than lesbians; and lesbians reported relying on friends for help and support more frequently than non-lesbians. Lesbians were more likely than non-lesbians to report expressing their anger; they reported less fighting spirit, less fatalism, and less cognitive avoidance than non-lesbians. Finally, Fobair et al. (2001) found lesbian women to be less satisfied with their physician's care and inclusion of their partner in medical treatment discussions than non-lesbians (as did Matthews et al., 2002).

Another recent study took a rather different approach to understanding the reactions of sexual minority women to breast cancer (Boehmer, Linde, & Freund, 2005). Rather than compare lesbians to heterosexual women, this study examined differences within a sample of 100 sexual minority women. The focus of the analyses was on the extent to which the women had previously disclosed their sexual orientation, and the way in which the women self-identified. This study found that women who self-identified as lesbians reported less distress than women who self-identified as bisexual or as partnered with women.

Research to date has provided important information, but it also has limitations. Boehme et al. (2005) did not compare the sexual minority women with heterosexual women. Matthews et al. (2002) had only 13 lesbian women in their sample, and the data were mostly qualitative. Fobair et al. (2001) did compare lesbians with heterosexuals, but there is no evidence that they tried to match the samples. The lesbian and heterosexual samples were similar in many respects, but they also differed in several respects. The lesbian sample was farther in time past their treatment than the heterosexual sample. The lesbians were also more educated, more likely to be professionally employed, less likely to be partnered, and less likely to have had children than the heterosexual women. There was no indication that these differences were controlled for in the analyses of outcome variables.

The present study adds to this accumulating information base, exploring similarities and differences between the psychosocial experience of lesbian and heterosexual women diagnosed with breast cancer. Due to the dearth of information available on this topic, we examined a number of variables, including choice of treatment (surgical and adjuvant), levels of distress and subjective quality of life, the finding of benefit in the cancer experience, a profile of the kinds of concerns for the future that the women hold, various kinds of variables bearing on the women's intimate relationship, several aspects of social support, and several aspects of coping. We did so in a sample of lesbian women and a sample of heterosexual women who were matched on age, ethnicity, and time since diagnosis, to minimize confounding effects of these variables between groups.

Although this study was in most respects exploratory, some tentative hypotheses were advanced. Following results of Kurdek (1988), we expected lesbians to report relying more on friends for support, whereas heterosexual women would report relying more on family. In line with the suggestion by Beren et al. (1996) that lesbian culture places less emphasis on the importance of physical appearance than does heterosexual culture, and the report by Kirkpatrick (1991) that lesbian culture values personal intimacy more than sex, we expected to see less concern about body-image and sexual issues among lesbian than heterosexual women. In line with the findings of Dibble and Roberts (2002), we did not expect to find differences in the types of medical treatment the groups of women received.

## *METHOD*

### Participants

All data collection for this study was approved by the University of Miami's Institutional Review Board: participants gave written informed consent before participating. Participants were 78 women diagnosed with early stage breast cancer. Of these, 39 were self-identified lesbians, recruited through a nationwide distribution of fliers via physicians, women's networks, and lesbian community resource centers. The fliers indicated that this project was examining the experience of adjusting to breast cancer diagnosis and treatment among lesbians. These lesbian participants then were matched by age, ethnicity, stage of disease, and approximate time since diagnosis to 39 self-identified heterosexual breast cancer patients. The latter were already participating in one of two other studies for which women were being recruited from several Miami-area hospitals and practices through fliers or letters sent to them by their physicians. These projects made no mention of interest in the experiences of lesbians, but they did assess sexual orientation as part of demographic assessment. Recruitment varied from near the time of diagnosis to 5 years after diagnosis and surgery.

Given these procedures, one difference between samples was built into the recruitment process: the lesbian women were from a broader geographic range than the heterosexual women, who were all from the Miami area. We had no specific eligibility criteria (other than self-reported sexual orientation for each subsample). Exclusion criteria included a previous diagnosis of cancer, advanced cancer (beyond Stage II), and psychopathology serious enough to have resulted in prior hospitalization.

### Data Collection

Data were collected by questionnaires that were sent to the women and returned by mail. Estimated time to complete measures was approximately an hour.

Several sorts of psychosocial measures were used in this research. They are grouped here in terms of measures that pertain to emotional well-being, measures that pertain to the woman's intimate relationship, and measures that pertain to social support resources and coping.

## Emotional Well-Being Measures

*Emotional distress.* One measure of emotional adjustment was the Center for Epidemiological Studies Depression scale (CES-D; Radloff, 1977). The CES-D is a 20-item scale assessing depressive symptomatology. Respondents indicated whether they have had a variety of experiences over the past week by answering a series of first-person sentences (e.g., "I felt I was just as good as other people"; "My sleep was restless"). Response options ranged from "Rarely or none of the time–less than 1 day" (0) to "most or all of the time–5-7 days" (3). Cronbach's alpha for this sample was .93 among lesbians, .95 among heterosexuals.

*Thought intrusion and avoidance.* Another measure bearing on distress was the Impact of Event Scale (IES; Horowitz et al., 1979). This measure has 15 items assessing participants' reactions to a stressful event (in this case, the diagnosis of breast cancer). Respondents indicated how frequently each statement has been true in the past 2 weeks. Response choices range from "not at all" (1) to "often" (4). The IES has two subscales: avoidance and intrusion. The avoidance subscale (8 items) assesses to what extent participants are actively avoiding thoughts about breast cancer. In this sample, Cronbach's alpha for this subscale was .69 among lesbians, .78 among heterosexuals. The intrusion subscale (7 items) assesses to what extent participants experience unwanted thoughts about breast cancer. Cronbach's alpha for this subscale was .87 among lesbians, .89 among heterosexuals.

*Perceived quality of life.* We also assessed participants' perceptions of their overall quality of life. Eleven items were selected from Andrews and Withey (1976), which address a reasonable range of life activities. Respondents considered each item's content and indicated how they felt about that domain of life, on a scale ranging from "terrible" (1) to "delighted" (7). Cronbach's alpha in this sample was .89 among lesbians, .94 among heterosexuals.

*Benefit finding.* Assessment in this study also included a measure of perceived benefits arising from the experience of diagnosis and treatment of breast cancer (Antoni et al., 2001; Tomich & Helgeson, 2004). The measure used in this study had 17 items. The stem for each was "Having had breast cancer has . . ." and the item expressed a potential benefit from the experience. Responses were made on a scale with labels "Not at all" (0), "A little" (1), "Moderately" (2), "Quite a bit" (3), and "Extremely" (4). The items assess benefits in a variety of domains, including acceptance of life's imperfections, becoming more cognizant of the role of other people in one's life, and developing a sense of purpose in life. Factor analysis suggests that the measure is appropriately used as a unitary scale (Urcuyo et al., 2005). Cronbach's alpha in this sample was .91 among lesbians, .93 among heterosexuals.

*Concerns about breast cancer.* Participants' concerns were assessed by two measures. The Profile of Concerns about Breast Cancer (PCBC) was developed by Spencer et al. (1999) to assess the concerns of breast cancer patients. The PCBC consists of 28 items, each naming a specific potential concern stemming from the diagnosis or medical treatment of breast cancer. Respondents were asked to rate on a scale of "not at all concerned" (0) to "extremely concerned" (4) how concerned they presently were about each individual issue.

Spencer et al. (1999) factor analyzed the 28 PCBC items and identified three factors: concerns about life and pain issues, concerns about rejection issues, and concerns about sexuality issues. Items about work, adjuvant treatment, and partner reactions were treated separately by Spencer et al. because the items did not apply to substantial numbers of patients. Within each of the latter categories the relevant items were highly correlated, however. As did Spencer et al., we examined the latter among the women to whom they were relevant. In this sample, Cronbach's alpha for the life and pain concern factor was .84 among lesbians, .86 among heterosexuals, and Cronbach's alpha for sexual concerns was .76 among lesbians, .91 among heterosexuals. In contrast to this similarity between groups on the first two factors, Cronbach's alpha for rejection concerns was .92 among heterosexuals but only .31 among lesbians. Given this very low alpha, this outcome variable was not examined further. Cronbach's alphas for work concern were .79 among lesbians and .85 among heterosexuals; for adjuvant treatment .87 among lesbians and .83 among heterosexuals; and for partner reaction .59 among lesbians and .69 among heterosexuals

*Concern about the body.* Another realm of concerns assessed here pertained to issues of appearance and body integrity. These concerns were conceptualized as individual differences in personality, and were assessed with the Measure of Body Apperception (MBA; Carver et al., 1998; Petronis et al., 2003). The MBA was designed to assess two aspects of women's concern about body image. These domains reflect the idea that feeling good about oneself depends on a sense of body integrity (4 items, e.g., "When something goes wrong inside your body, you're never really the same person again") and the idea that feeling good about oneself depends on appearance (4 items, e.g., "I feel good about myself only if I know I look good to other people"). Respondents rated each statement from "strongly agree" (1) to "strongly disagree" (4). Cronbach's alpha for investment in body integrity in this sample was .55 among lesbians, .66 among heterosexuals; Cronbach's alpha for investment in physical appearance was .84 among lesbians, .67 among heterosexuals. Although the alpha for investment in body integrity among lesbians was low (even for this small number of items), we did go on to examine group differences on this characteristic.

## Relationship-Related Measures

*Relationship satisfaction.* Relationship satisfaction was assessed by an item from the Quality of Marriage Index (QMI; Norton, 1983). The item was a rating of the extent of the woman's overall satisfaction with the relationship, on a 7-point scale, with response options ranging from "extremely unhappy" (1) to "extreme joy" (7).

*Perceptions of partner reactions.* A set of ad hoc items was included to measure the woman's perceptions of her partner's reaction to her diagnosis and surgery. These items assess the woman's perception of how bothered the partner is by the surgical scar; the degree to which the partner is currently expressing affection to her; the extent to which the couple is experiencing friction between them; and how the partner is reacting to the idea that cancer represents a threat to the participant's life (ranging from distancing to holding on closely).

*Sexual disruption.* Disruption in the sexual aspect of the relationship was assessed by the Sexual Relations subscale from the Psychosocial Adjustment to Illness Scale (PAIS), a self-report measure of how illness is influencing well-being more broadly (Derogatis, 1975). The six Sexual Relations items assess changes in sexual interest, activities, and abilities. Each item has its own response options. Cronbach's alpha for this sample was .76 among lesbians, .69 among heterosexuals.

*Sexual activity.* Specific items were included in the assessment protocol to measure the frequency of sexual relations, the participants' reported level of satisfaction with the sexual aspects of the relationship, and the extent to which the participant versus the partner initiates sexual relations. Responses to the latter item ranged from "my partner initiates sexual activity hardly at all" (1) through "my partner initiates sexual activity about as often as I do" (3) to "my partner initiates sexual activity almost always" (5). These items were completed with respect to the current situation and also retrospectively with regard to the situation as it existed before the cancer diagnosis.

*Psychosexual adjustment.* What we refer to here as psychosexual adjustment was a set of items selected by Carver et al. (1998) from previous studies of the impact of mastectomy versus lumpectomy. These are self-ratings of attractiveness ("How physically attractive do you feel you are?"), sexual desirability ("How sexually desirable do you feel you are?"), femininity ("How feminine, or how much like a woman, do you feel you are?"), sexual inhibition ("How sexually inhibited do you feel you are?"), and perceived change in sense of self ("To what extent do you feel not like yourself anymore"?). Items were rated on scales ranging from "not at all" (0) to "extremely" (4). Analyses were conducted on each item individually.

## Social Support and Coping

Two aspects of dealing with stressful experiences that are widely regarded as important are the social support resources the person has and the coping reactions that emerge in response to the stressor. These variables were also assessed in this study.

*Social support.* We measured both received social support and perceived social support. The Social Network Scale (SNS; Lubben, 1988) is a brief, 10-item scale that has been widely used with diverse populations and measures the frequency of contact with friends and relatives. This measure was not used as a total score in this study. Rather, because we had hypotheses about the relative role of friends and family in the support networks of the two groups under study, specific items pertaining to friends and family were examined separately.

Perceived availability of overall social support was measured using a brief scale (6 items) derived from the Interpersonal Support Evaluation List (ISEL; Cohen, Mermelstein, Kamrack, & Hoberman, 1985), a widely used measure with high internal consistency. The ISEL was designed to assess the perceived availability of social support in four domains, tangible or material aid, belonging or people to do things with, self-esteem or a positive comparison when comparing oneself to others, and appraisal or someone with whom to talk about ones problems. The version used here had at least one item from each of the four domains. Cronbach's alpha for this sample was .74 among lesbians, .86 among heterosexuals.

Due to a difference in questionnaires administered to participants who were more than 16 months past their surgery, social support variables could be explored in only a subset of the total sample. Those analyses pertain to 26 lesbians and 26 heterosexual women.

*Coping.* Several aspects of coping responses were assessed by the Brief COPE (Carver, 1997). The scales of the Brief COPE include acceptance, active coping, planning, behavioral disengagement, denial, substance use, humor, positive reframing, religious coping, self-distraction, use of emotional support from friends, use of emotional support from partner, and venting. Each scale has two items. Participants were told to rate how often they used the response in trying to deal with the stresses related to their diagnosis and surgery. The answer choices ranged from "I haven't been doing this at all" (0) to "I've been doing this a lot" (3). Scales were scored (separately) by averaging the relevant item responses.

## Data Analysis

Preliminary analyses determined that matching of the samples on age, ethnicity, and time since diagnosis did not produce associations on outcome variables at a level greater than chance. Thus the subsamples were treated as independent. Data analysis began by examining medical and demographic variables that might have to be controlled statistically in comparisons of psychosocial variables (which were our main focus); variables were included if they both differed between groups and related to the psychosocial variables at $p < .05$. Those initial comparisons were by *t* test for continuous variables and chi-square for categorical variables. The subsequent comparisons on the psychosocial variables of interest were by analysis of covariance, controlling for medical and demographic variables identified as differing between groups. We tested whether correlations between distress and the other psychosocial variables differed significantly from one group to the other, using z tests to compare correlations. Finally, for measures in which we asked for retrospective ratings as well as current status, we conducted repeated-measures analysis of covariance (crossed by group). Because our purpose here was exploratory, all tests used a .05 significance criterion.

## RESULTS

### Sample Information

Table 1 contains comparisons of demographic and medical variables between lesbian and non-lesbian subsamples. Fewer lesbians received radiation therapy than heterosexuals, and lesbians had significantly

TABEL 1. Comparisons Between Lesbian and Heterosexual Breast Cancer Patients on Demographic and Medical Variables.

| | Lesbian (n = 39) M (SD) | Heterosexual (n = 39) M (SD) | Statistic | p |
|---|---|---|---|---|
| Age (years) | 48.33 (8.26) | 49.41 (8.89) | t = .55 | .58 |
| Education (years) | 16.97 (2.88) | 15.10 (2.27) | t = 3.19 | .01 |
| Ethnicity | | | | |
| Non-Hispanic White | 36 (92.3%) | 29 (74.4%) | | |
| Black | 1 (2.6%) | 6 (15.4%) | | |
| Hispanic | 2 (5.1%) | 4 (10.2%) | $\chi^2$ = 4.99 | .08 |
| Relationship status | | | | |
| Married/Partnered | 24 (61.5%) | 26 (66.7%) | | |
| Separated/Divorced | 3 (7.7%) | 9 (23.0%) | | |
| Single | 12 (30.8%) | 4 (10.3%) | $\chi^2$ = 7.19 | .07 |
| Relationship length (months)[†] | 68.69 (60.80) | 198.87 (158.55) | t = 4.17 | .01 |
| Employment status | | | | |
| Employed | 28 (71.8%) | 31 (79.4) | | |
| Not employed | 11 (28.2%) | 8 (20.5) | $\chi^2$ = .64 | .73 |
| Months since surgery | 17.21 (16.92) | 17.33 (16.71) | t = .03 | .97 |
| Disease stage | | | | |
| Stage 0 | 4 (10.3%) | 3 (7.7%) | | |
| Stage I | 22 (56.4%) | 24 (61.5%) | | |
| Stage II | 13 (33.3%) | 12 (30.8%) | $\chi^2$ = .27 | .84 |
| Positive lymph nodes | 1.97 (5.70) | 0.85 (3.02) | t = 1.09 | .28 |
| Surgical procedure | | | | |
| Mastectomy | 25 (64.1%) | 18 (46.2%) | | |
| Lumpectomy | 14 (35.9%) | 12 (30.8%) | $\chi^2$ = 2.54 | .11 |
| Chemotherapy | 19 (48.7%) | 15 (38.5%) | $\chi^2$ = .83 | .36 |
| Radiation | 13 (33.3%) | 23 (59.0%) | $\chi^2$ = 5.16 | .02 |
| Anti-hormonal | 14 (35.9%) | 10 (25.6%) | $\chi^2$ = 1.13 | .29 |
| Reconstruction | 7 (17.9%) | 12 (30.8%) | $\chi^2$ = 1.74 | .19 |

[†] This variable pertains only to the subsample who reported being partnered.

more education than heterosexuals. Accordingly, education and radiation were controlled in all subsequent analyses. Among participants in relationships, lesbians reported significantly shorter relationship length than heterosexuals. This variable was controlled in analyses of relationship-related outcomes.

## Emotional Well-Being

Comparisons between the groups on measures reflecting emotional adjustment are shown in Table 2. Lesbians reported significantly less active avoidance of thoughts about cancer than heterosexual women, *though they* did not differ in reports of thought intrusions. Heterosexual women reported considerably more benefit from the breast cancer experience than did lesbians. Heterosexual women reported significantly higher levels of concern about sexual issues than did lesbian women.

Another area of potential concern in dealing with breast cancer is body image, both in the form of the sense of body integrity and in the form of physical appearance. Heterosexual women reported greater concern about their appearance on the MBA than did lesbian women but the groups did not differ on concerns about body integrity.

## Relationship-Related Measures

Various aspects of the participants' intimate relationships were also explored. These are summarized in Table 3. As noted earlier, only the women who reported being in partnered relationships completed measures pertaining to the relationship. Only those who reported being in sexual relationships reported on the measures pertaining to sexual activity.

The groups did not differ on relationship satisfaction nor did they differ in reports of how bothered they thought their partners were by their surgical scar, how much affection their partners were demonstrating toward them, whether there was increased fighting or friction between the couple, or how their partners were reacting to breast cancer as a threat to their life.

On the sexual disruption subscale from the PAIS, heterosexual women reported that there had been more disruption in their sexual relationship since their diagnosis and treatment than did lesbians. Lesbians tended to report having engaged in sexual activity less frequently before diagnosis than heterosexuals, though the difference fell just short of statistical significance. However, repeated measures ANCOVA (controlling for education, radiation, and relationship length), indicated that reported

TABLE 2. Comparisons Between Lesbian and Heterosexual Breast Cancer Patients on Measures Relating to Emotional Well-Being.

| | Lesbian (n = 39) M (SD) | Heterosexual (n = 39) M (SD) | Statistic | p |
|---|---|---|---|---|
| CES-D[1] | 11.89 (2.11) | 15.80 (2.11) | F = 1.58 | .21 |
| IES[2] avoidance | 1.65 (.10) | 2.05 (.10) | F = 7.28 | .01 |
| IES intrusion | 2.11 (.14) | 2.45 (.14) | F = 2.76 | .10 |
| Perceived quality of life | 4.60 (.17) | 4.51 (.17) | F = 0.12 | .73 |
| Benefit finding | 31.60 (2.24) | 43.67 (2.21) | F = 13.50 | .001 |
| PCBC[3] life and pain concerns | 2.52 (.14) | 2.50 (.15) | F = 0.01 | .93 |
| PCBC sexual concerns | 1.91 (.19) | 2.53 (.19) | F = 4.36 | .04 |
| PCBC work concern items[†] | 2.01 (.22) | 1.85 (.22) | F = 0.24 | .62 |
| PCBC adjuv-treatment concern items[†] | 3.54 (.24) | 3.67 (.23) | F = 0.14 | .71 |
| PCBC partner reaction concern items[†] | 2.20 (.19) | 2.36 (.20) | F = 1.49 | .57 |
| MBA[4] body integrity concerns | 9.04 (.53) | 9.47 (.53) | F = 0.31 | .58 |
| MBA physical appearance concerns | 7.63 (.55) | 9.70 (.55) | F = 6.62 | .01 |

NOTE: Means are adjusted for radiation treatment and education.
[†] These items were completed only by those women to whom they were relevant.
[1] Center for Epidemiological Studies Depression Scale
[2] Impact of Event Scale
[3] Profile of Concerns about Breast Cancer
[4] Measure of Body Apperception

sexual frequency did not change significantly overall from pre-diagnosis to post-surgery. Nor did sexual frequency over time interact significantly with sexual orientation (p = .15).

Lesbian and heterosexual women did not differ in reported sexual satisfaction before diagnosis. Repeated measures ANCOVA indicated that sexual satisfaction did not change significantly overall from pre-diagnosis to post-diagnosis, nor did change over time interact significantly with sexual orientation (p = .59). Heterosexual women (more than lesbians) reported retrospectively that their partners initiated sexual activity more frequently than they did themselves before the cancer diagnosis. This difference was not quite significant at the time of assessment (p = .06). A repeated measures analysis showed that reports of initiation of sexual activity did not change significantly from pre-diag-

TABLE 3. Comparisons Between Lesbian and Heterosexual Breast Cancer Patients on Relationship-Related Variables.

| | Lesbian M (SD) | Heterosexual M (SD) | Statistic | p |
|---|---|---|---|---|
| | (n = 25) | (n = 25) | | |
| Relationship satisfaction | 3.65 (.44) | 3.43 (.44) | F = 0.11 | .74 |
| How bothered is partner by scar | 1.67 (.20) | 1.66 (.20) | F = 0.00 | .97 |
| Partner expressing affection | 4.24 (.21) | 4.08 (.21) | F = 0.23 | .63 |
| Fighting/friction | 1.75 (.20) | 1.75 (.19) | F = 0.00 | 1.00 |
| Partner reaction to threat to life | 2.03 (.23) | 2.25 (.22) | F = 0.40 | .53 |
| | (n = 28) | (n = 28) | | |
| PAIS[1] sexual disruption | 1.62 (.12) | 2.02 (.12) | F = 4.44 | .04 |
| Sexual frequency pre-surgery | 4.30 (1.03) | 7.10 (.97) | F = 3.29 | .07 |
| Sexual frequency at assessment | 4.09 (1.17) | 3.87 (1.17) | F = 0.15 | .70 |
| Sexual satisfaction pre-surgery | 3.89 (.21) | 3.97 (.20) | F = 0.73 | .79 |
| Sexual satisfaction at assessment | 3.36 (.29) | 3.14 (.29) | F = 0.06 | .80 |
| Partner initiated sex pre-surgery | 2.84 (.24) | 3.74 (.22) | F = 6.39 | .01 |
| Partner initiated sex at assessment | 2.65 (.29) | 3.14 (.28) | F = 3.84 | .06 |
| | (n = 39) | (n = 39) | | |
| How physically attractive do you feel | 2.81 (.18) | 2.75 (.18) | F = 0.05 | .82 |
| How feminine do you feel | 3.24 (.20) | 3.13 (.19) | F = 0.17 | .68 |
| How sexually desirable do you feel | 2.98 (.19) | 2.66 (.19) | F = 1.42 | .24 |
| How much "not like yourself anymore" | 2.05 (.22) | 2.58 (.23) | F = 2.04 | .16 |

NOTE: Means are adjusted for radiation, education, and relationship length.
[1] Psychosocial Adjustment to Illness Scale

nosis to post-diagnosis, nor did sexual initiative over time interact with sexual orientation (p = .22).

## Social Support and Coping

Lesbians and heterosexual women did not differ significantly in their reports of perceived available social support on the brief ISEL (Table 4).

TABLE 4. Comparisons Between Lesbian and Heterosexual Breast Cancer Patients on Aspects of Social Support and Coping.

| | Lesbian M (SD) | Heterosexual M (SD) | Statistic | p |
|---|---|---|---|---|
| | (n = 26) | (n = 26) | | |
| Overall perceived social support (ISEL[1]) | 21.32 (.64) | 21.34 (.63) | F = 0.00 | .98 |
| Number relatives seen monthly (SNS[2]) | 2.32 (.22) | 3.42 (.22) | F = 11.66 | .001 |
| Number close relatives (SNS) | 1.87 (.26) | 2.81 (.25) | F = 6.10 | .02 |
| Number friends seen monthly (SNS) | 3.32 (.22) | 2.93 (.21) | F = 1.51 | .23 |
| Number of close friends (SNS) | 3.55 (.22) | 3.08 (.21) | F = 2.21 | .14 |
| | (n = 39) | (n = 39) | | |
| Active coping | 2.83 (.17) | 2.76 (.17) | F = 0.06 | .80 |
| Self distraction | 2.21 (.13) | 2.41 (.13) | F = 1.02 | .32 |
| Denial | 1.21 (.11) | 1.63 (.12) | F = 6.18 | .01 |
| Substance Use | 1.46 (.12) | 1.16 (.14) | F = 2.46 | .12 |
| Use of emotional support from friends | 3.19 (.16) | 2.70 (.16) | F = 4.11 | .05 |
| Use of emotional support from partner | 2.63 (.21) | 2.57 (.21) | F = 0.03 | .86 |
| Behavioral disengagement | 1.20 (.09) | 1.24 (.10) | F = 0.08 | .78 |
| Venting | 2.51 (.13) | 2.07 (.14) | F = 4.75 | .03 |
| Positive Reframing | 2.98 (.15) | 2.43 (.15) | F = 5.98 | .02 |
| Planning | 2.82 (.17) | 2.36 (.18) | F = 3.46 | .07 |
| Humor | 2.24 (.15) | 1.94 (.16) | F = 1.74 | .19 |
| Acceptance | 3.41 (.13) | 3.09 (.13) | F = 2.80 | .10 |
| Religion | 2.35 (.16) | 2.45 (.16) | F = 0.19 | .67 |

NOTE: Means are adjusted for radiation and education.
[1] Interpersonal Support Evaluation List
[2] Social Network Scale

Regarding specific aspects of social network assessed with individual items from the SNS, two differences emerged. Heterosexual women reported being in at least monthly contact with a larger number of relatives than did lesbians. Heterosexual women also reported having a larger number of relatives than lesbian women to whom they felt close and at ease talking about private matters or asking for help.

Lesbian and heterosexual women differed significantly in their use of several coping strategies (Table 4). Heterosexual women reported engaging in denial more than did lesbian women. On the other hand, lesbians used emotional support from friends, positive reframing, and venting to a greater degree than did heterosexual women. Lesbian women also tended to endorse planning more, but this tendency fell just short of statistical significance.

## Relationship Between Depressive Symptoms and Other Variables

We then examined relationships between reported levels of depressive symptoms (from CES-D scores) and other variables assessed. We did this by comparing the correlations that were found within the two groups to each other by z test. Correlations differed significantly between groups in only one case. Concerns about body integrity related more closely to distress among lesbians ($r = .56$) than among heterosexual women ($r = .08$), $z = 2.03$, $p < .05$. (Indeed, the relation of concern about body integrity to depression among lesbians was fully as strong as the internal reliability of the MBA scale itself in that group.) Relationships between distress and coping were also explored, in the same manner. The reaction of behavioral disengagement related more closely to CES-D scores among heterosexual women ($r = .69$) than among lesbians ($r = -.01$), $z = 3.36$, $p < .01$.

## DISCUSSION

Several aspects of the experience of dealing with a diagnosis of early stage breast cancer were explored among lesbian and matched heterosexual women who had had surgery for breast cancer from 2 to 62 months previously. We compared the groups on psychological variables, controlling for demographic and medical variables that differentiated the groups (education level, treatment with radiation, and length of relationship).

## Emotional Well-Being

Depressive symptomatology was low overall and, as expected, reported depressive symptoms did not differ significantly between lesbians and heterosexuals. Nor did the groups differ in reported amount of intrusive thoughts about the breast cancer experience, as measured by the IES. However, in several ways the reactions of lesbians seemed muted, compared to those of heterosexual women. One example occurred on the second IES subscale. Lesbians reported significantly less effort to avoid thoughts about breast cancer than did heterosexuals (as was also found by Fobair et al., 2001). It is plausible (though speculative) that persons who are accustomed to dealing with stressors make less effort to avoid thoughts about them. Perhaps lesbians are less in need of such a defense, having dealt with additional stressors in the process of coming to terms with their sexuality.

The muted response of lesbians also appeared on a measure of having derived benefit from the experience of dealing with cancer. Lesbians reported substantially less benefit finding than did the heterosexual sample, though they reported no difference in satisfaction with their lives on another measure. Again, one might speculate on the basis of other literature concerning benefit finding (Antoni et al., 2001; Urcuyo et al., 2005) that the lesbian sample, in the course of living as a minority in a hostile environment, may already have faced multiple challenges, and that the diagnosis of breast cancer may represent just one more in a series of opportunities for growth. For heterosexuals, on the other hand, being diagnosed with a life-threatening illness may have been the first major instance of adversity prompting such soul searching.

### Sexuality

Another area in which the responses of the lesbian sample seemed more muted than those of the heterosexual sample was issues concerning sexuality. Heterosexual women reported more concerns about sexual issues on the PCBC, compared to lesbians. They also reported having greater concern about (or investment in) their appearance on the MBA than did lesbians (though no difference emerged regarding concern about body integrity). These findings seem consistent with Kirkpatrick's (1991) report that closeness is valued more than sex in lesbian relationships and Beren et al.'s (1996) suggestion that lesbian culture places less emphasis than heterosexual culture on the importance of physical appearance. Thus, concerns about sexual issues and issues of appearance would not be as salient for lesbian women as for heterosexuals.

The sexual aspect of their relationships was also explored more directly. Consistent with the literature suggesting that sexual frequency tends to be lower in lesbians couples (Herbert, 1996), lesbians exhibited a marginal tendency to report lower frequency of sex, before being diagnosed with breast cancer. This difference was not maintained, however, at the time of assessment. Lesbians also reported less disruption in their sexual relationship since diagnosis than was reported by hetero-sexuals. This finding is, again, consistent with the idea that less empha-sis is placed on sex in lesbian relationships as compared to heterosexual relationships (Kirkpatrick, 1991; Herbert, 1996).

Consistent with the description of lesbian relationship roles as more egalitarian (Klinger, 1996), heterosexuals (more than lesbians) reported that their partners initiated sexual activity more frequently than they did themselves before the cancer diagnosis and tended to report the same post-surgery. Also consistent with the literature (Klinger, 1996), length of relationships was significantly shorter among lesbian than among heterosexuals in this study. Although groups were expected to differ in reported partner reactions and relationship friction, no significant dif-ference was noted between groups in those respects.

## Coping

Also explored in this study were mechanisms of coping reported by the women. Heterosexual women reported engaging in denial (an overt pushing away of the experience) more than lesbian women. Lesbians, on the other hand, relied on emotional support from friends, positive reframing, and venting their feelings more than did heterosexuals. Overall, lesbians appeared to employ more adaptive forms of coping. This is consistent both with the higher level of education among lesbi-ans (although education was controlled for in these comparisons) and with the fact that, just by virtue of being a minority group, lesbians may have had to cope with challenging situation more frequently than non-lesbians over the course of their lives and may thus have had more op-portunities to learn adaptive forms of coping (see also Roberts, 2001).

The pattern of coping found here resembles that reported by Fobair et al. (2001) in several respects, though the studies used different mea-sures. Fobair et al. found that lesbians were more likely than heterosex-uals to report expressions of their anger (which is akin to venting from the Brief COPE). They also found that lesbians were less likely to report fighting spirit and fatalism and non-significant tendency for lesbians to engage in less cognitive avoidance (the latter of which is akin to denial from the Brief COPE) was observed.

## Sources of Support

It has been argued that lesbians do not differ from heterosexual women in the amount of their overall social support, but that the groups tend to draw their support from different sources (Kurdek, 1987, 1988).

Specifically, it is argued that lesbian women frequently have a tenuous relationship with their families of origin, and that it is common for lesbians to select "families of choice" composed of close friends. Consistent with this general line of reasoning, lesbians and heterosexuals in this study did not differ significantly in their reports of overall support they perceived as available, on the measure derived from the ISEL.

However, when asked to indicate how many family members they were in frequent contact with and how many family members they felt close to and at ease talking with about private matters or asking for help, lesbians reported lower numbers than did heterosexual women (consistent with results of Fobair et al., 2001). No such difference emerged when they were asked the same questions about friends, however. Indeed, when indicating how they had been coping with the stresses associated with the cancer diagnosis and treatment, lesbians were more likely than heterosexual women to report that they had been obtaining support from their friends.

### *Limitations*

We should also point explicitly to several limitations in the study. We used samples of convenience, which potentially introduce recruitment and selection bias arising from the use of volunteer participants. Thus, the extent of generalizability to broader populations is unknown. We tried to match each lesbian participant (who were less readily recruited) with a heterosexual participant on several characteristics. However, we were not fully successful in doing so. Both groups were relatively highly educated, but they differed significantly in that regard, with more education among the lesbians. Another limitation was that a number of other variables might have been as important in matching, as well, which we did not assess. As noted earlier the groups differed geographically: the lesbian women were recruited through a nationwide network of contacts, whereas the heterosexual women all were residents of south Florida. The consequences of these differences are unknown. Finally, the sample was not as large as would be desirable. Given the limited statistical power of the study and the large number of analyses conducted, which could have resulted in statistical significance occurring by chance, the results should be interpreted with caution.

### *Future Directions*

Although findings are generally consistent among the studies available on the experience of lesbians with breast cancer, there is much yet to be learned before adequate mental health care can be provided to this population. As in any culture, heterogeneity within the group is as prevalent as differences between groups. Therefore, findings must always be interpreted with caution and used as guideposts to detect issues that warrant attention. As social support and the relative role of friends versus family appear to function differently for lesbians and heterosexual women, future work should further explore the various types and sources of support. Our data also suggests that lesbians and heterosexuals cope somewhat differently. As coping skills training is an integral part of most psychosocial interventions for breast cancer, it is imperative that these differences be explored further. Although much remains to be explored, the ever-increasing awareness of and interest in minority issues in mental health provides hope for the future.

# REFERENCES

American Cancer Society website (*www.cancer.org*) (2005).

Andrews, F. M., & Withey, S. B. (1976). *Social indicators of well being: Americans' perceptions of life quality*. New York: Plenum.

Antoni, M. H., Lehman, J. M., Kilbourn, K. M., Boyers, A. E., Culver, J. L., Alferi, S. M., Yount, S. E., McGregor, B. A., Arena, P. L., Harris, S. D., Price, A. A. & Carver, C. S. (2001). Cognitive-behavioral stress management intervention decreases the prevalence of depression and enhances benefit finding among women under treatment for early-stage breast cancer. *Health Psychology, 20*, 20-32.

Beren, S. E., Hayden, H. A., Wilfley, D. E., & Grilo, C. M. (1996). The influence of sexual orientation on body dissatisfaction in adult men and women. *International Journal of Eating Disorders, 20*, 135-141.

Boehmer, U., Linde, R., & Freund, K. M. (2005). Sexual minority women's coping and psychological adjustment after a diagnosis of breast cancer. *Journal of Women's Health, 14*, 214-224.

Carver, C. S. (1997). You want to measure coping but your protocol's too long: Consider the Brief COPE. *International Journal of Behavioral Medicine, 4*, 92-100.

Carver, C. S., Pozo, C., Harris, S. D., Noriega, V, Scheier, M. F., Robinson, D. S., Ketcham, A. S., Moffat, F. L. & Clark, K. C. (1993). How coping mediates the effect of optimism on distress: A study of women with early stage breast cancer. *Journal of Personality and Social Psychology, 65*, 375-390.

Carver, C.S., Pozo-Kaderman, C., Price, A.A., Noriega, V., Harris, S.D., Derhagopian, R.P., Robinson, D.S., & Moffatt, Jr., F.L. (1998). Concern about aspects of body image and adjustment to early stage breast cancer. *Psychosomatic Medicine, 60*, 168-174.

Culver, J. L., Arena, P. L., Antoni, M. H., & Carver, C. S. (2002). Coping and distress among women under treatment for early stage breast cancer: Comparing African Americans, Hispanics, and non-Hispanic Whites. *Psycho-Oncology, 11*, 495-504.

Culver, J. L., Arena, P. L., Wimberly, S. R., Antoni, M. H., & Carver, C. S. (2004). Coping among African American, Hispanic, and non-Hispanic White women recently treated for early stage breast cancer. *Psychology and Health, 19,* 157-166.

Derogatis, L. R. (1975). *The Psychosocial Adjustment to Illness Scale: Administration, scoring, and procedures manual.* Baltimore, MD: Johns Hopkins University Press.

Dibble, S. L., & Roberts, S. A. (2002). A comparison of breast cancer diagnosis and treatment between lesbian and heterosexual women. *Journal of the Gay and Lesbian Medical Association, 6,* 9-16.

Fobair, P., O'Hanlan, K., Koopman, C., Classen, C., Dimiceli, S., Drooker, N., Warner, D., Davis, H. R., Loulan, J., Wallsten, D., Goffinet, D., Morrow, G., & Spiegel, D. (2001). Comparisons of lesbian and heterosexual women's response to newly diagnosed breast cancer. *Psycho-Oncology, 10,* 40-51.

Glanz, K. & Lerman, C. (1992). Psychosocial impact of breast cancer: A critical review. *Annals of Behavioral Medicine, 14,* 204-212.

Herbert, S. E. (1996). Lesbian sexuality. In Cabaj, R. P. & Stein, T. S. (Eds.), *Textbook of homosexuality and mental health.* (pp. 723-742). Washington, DC: American Psychiatric Press.

Horowitz, M., Wilner, N., & Alvarez, W. (1979). Impact of events scale. *Psychosomatic Medicine, 41,* 209-218.

Kirkpatrick, M. (1991). Lesbian couples in therapy. *Psychiatric Annals, 21,* 491-496.

Klinger, R. L. (1996). Lesbian couples. In Cabaj, R. P. & Stein, T. S. (Eds.), *Textbook of homosexuality and mental health.* (pp. 339-352). Washington, DC: American Psychiatric Press.

Kurdek, L. (1988). Perceived social support in gays and lesbians in cohabitating relationships. *Journal of Personality and Social Psychology, 54,* 504-509.

Kurdek, L. & Schmitt, P. (1986). Relationship quality of partners in heterosexual married, heterosexual cohabiting, and gay and lesbian relationships. *Journal of Personality and Social Psychology, 51,* 711-720.

Kurdek, L. & Schmitt, J. P. (1987). Perceived emotional support from family and friends in members of homosexual, married, and heterosexual cohabiting couples. *Journal of Homosexualtiy, 14,* 57-68.

Lubben, J.E. (1988). Assessing social networks among elderly populations. *Family and Community-Health, 11*(3), 42-52.

Matthews, A. K., Peterman, A. H., Delaney, P., Menard, L., & Brandenburg, D. (2002). A qualitative exploration of the experiences of lesbian and heterosexual patients with breast cancer. *Oncology Nursing Forum, 29,* 1455-1462.

McNair, D. M., Lorr, M. & Droppleman, L. F. (1971/1981). *Profile of mood states manual.* San Diego, CA: Educational & Industrial Testing Services.

Moyer, A. & Salovey, P. (1996). Psychosocial sequelae of breast cancer and its treatment. *Annals of Behavioral Medicine, 18,* 110-125.

Norton, R. (1983). Measuring marital quality: A critical look at the dependent variable. *Journal of Marriage and the Family, 45,* 141-151.

Petronis, V.M., Carver, C. S., Antoni, M. H., Weiss, S. (2003). Investment in body image and psychosocial well-being among women treated for early stage breast cancer: Partial replication and extension. *Psychology and Health, 18,* 1-13.

Radloff, L.S. (1977). The CES-D scale: A self-report depression scale for research in the general population. *Applied Psychological Measurement, 1*, 385-401.

Roberts, S. J. (2001). Lesbian health research: A review and recommendations for future research. *Health Care For Women International, 22*, 537-552.

Spencer, S. M., Lehman, J. L., Wynings, C., Arena, P., Carver, C. S., Antoni, M. H., Derhagopian, R. P., Ironson, G., Love, N. (1999). Concerns about breast cancer and relations to psychosocial well-being in a multi-ethnic sample of early stage patients. *Health Psychology, 18*, 159-168.

Tomich, P. L., Helgeson, V. S. (2004). Is finding something good in the bad always good? Benefit finding among women with breast cancer. *Health Psychology, 23*, 16-23.

Urcuyo, K. R., Boyers, A. E., Carver, C. S., & Antoni, M. H. (2005). Finding benefit in breast cancer: Relations with personality, coping, and concurrent well-being. *Psychology and Health, 20*, 175-192.

Williamson, G. M. (2000). Extending the activity restriction model of depressed affect: Evidence from a sample of breast cancer patients. *Health Psychology, 19*, 339-347.

doi:10.1300/J013v44n02_05

# Consequences
# of Frequenting the Lesbian Bar

Elisabeth Gruskin, DrPH
Kimberly Byrne, EdD
Susan Kools, RN, PhD
Andrea Altschuler, PhD

**SUMMARY.** Research indicates that lesbians who frequent bars are more likely to drink and that lesbians drink more than their heterosexual counterparts. We explored in detail the consequences of lesbians' bar attendance. We conducted 35 in-person, semi-structured interviews and analyzed the data using qualitative methods. The findings are organized

Elisabeth Gruskin and Andrea Altschuler are affiliated with Kaiser Permanente Division of Research, 2000 Broadway, Oakland, CA 94612.

Kimberly Byrne is affiliated with the Community Led Evaluation and Research, 1551 Madison Street, #210, Oakland, CA 94612.

Susan Kools is affiliated with the University of California San Francisco, San Francisco, CA 94143.

Address correspondence to: Elisabeth Gruskin, DrPH, Kaiser Permanente Division of Research, 2000 Broadway, Oakland, CA 94612 (E-mail: lpg@dor.kaiser.org).

Dr. Gruskin thanks her classmates in the qualitative courses at the University of California at San Francisco Nursing Program for their assistance with analyses of this study. The authors greatly appreciate the feedback from Andy Avins, Laura Enriquez, Joanne Gruskin, Joe Selby, and Carol Somkin on earlier drafts.

This project was funded by Kaiser Permanente and by the National Institute of Alcohol Abuse and Alcoholism K01 #AA13390.

An earlier version of this paper was presented as a poster session at the International Society of Addictive Medicine in Helsinki, Finland.

[Haworth co-indexing entry note]: "Consequences of Frequenting the Lesbian Bar." Gruskin, Elisabeth et al. Co-published simultaneously in *Women & Health* (The Haworth Medical Press, an imprint of The Haworth Press, Inc.) Vol. 44, No. 2, 2006, pp. 103-120; and: *Preventive Health Measures for Lesbian and Bisexual Women* (ed: Shelly Kerr, and Robin Mathy) The Haworth Medical Press, an imprint of The Haworth Press, Inc., 2006, pp. 103-120. Single or multiple copies of this article are available for a fee from The Haworth Document Delivery Service [1-800-HAWORTH, 9:00 a.m. - 5:00 p.m. (EST). E-mail address: docdelivery@haworthpress.com].

Available online at http://wh.haworthpress.com
doi:10.1300/J013v44n02_06

into the following categories: safety and support over the life course; lesbian identity development; reduction of stress; and social networks and intimate relationships. In each category, participants' stories are presented to highlight the health tradeoffs associated with bar patronage, the psychosocial importance of the bar, and the relationship between minority stress and alcohol use. Public health implications are discussed. doi:10.1300/J013v44n02_06 *[Article copies available for a fee from The Haworth Document Delivery Service: 1-800-HAWORTH. E-mail address: <docdelivery@haworthpress.com> Website: <http://www.HaworthPress.com> © 2006 by The Haworth Press, Inc. All rights reserved.]*

**KEYWORDS.** Alcohol, bars, lesbians, alcohol problems, substance abuse

## *INTRODUCTION*

*Jane, study participant, 37 years*

> I loved spending time in lesbian bars, because it was the only place I felt I could just be who I was. I could be affectionate with women. I could be gay . . . Nobody was going to talk about me . . . I mean, it was just a place where you felt free . . . In bars, you're beautiful. Everybody loves you, and you can be gay, and you can be whatever. In the real world, that's not the case.

The lesbian bar has been a cornerstone of lesbian culture since the 1920s (Faderman, 1991), and even today, lesbians continue to frequent these establishments to fulfill a wide range of needs with varying health consequences. Prior to the 1970s, women experienced harassment and violence at lesbian bars (Faderman, 1991). However, the social milieu of lesbian bars is attractive enough for lesbians to risk these negative consequences to meet their needs for social connection (Faderman, 1991; Wolfe, 1997). Recent studies confirm that bars remain an important social space for lesbians (Parks, 1999b; Wolfe, 1997).

Studies link alcohol use and frequenting lesbian bars (Heffernan, 1998; Parks, 1999b; Bloomfield, 1993). According to a limited number of studies, lesbians' drinking is similar to heterosexuals' drinking (Bloomfield, 1993). However, most recent studies found that lesbians consume more alcohol than heterosexual women (Aaron et al., 2001; Bergmark, 1999; Cochran et al., 2000; Diamant et al., 2000; Drabble et al., 2005; Gruskin et al., 2001; Mays et al., 2002; Nawyn et al., 2000; Skinner & Otis, 1996). In addition, Bergmark (1999), Diamant et al. (2000), and Drabble et al. (2005) found that lesbians were less likely to abstain from alcohol than their heterosexual counterparts. Lesbians also reported higher rates of alcohol problems and/or negative consequences (Cochran et al., 2000; Dibble et al., 2004; Drabble et al., 2005; Gilman et al., 2001; Hughes, 2003) and alcohol dependence than heterosexual women.

Several researchers have hypothesized that lesbians' higher levels of alcohol consumption and abuse can be attributed to the high levels of stress caused by the discrimination and marginalization in society that lesbians experience. Nawyn et al. (2000) found a link between workplace harassment and increased alcohol consumption and problems for lesbians. Heffernan (1998) found that lesbians' perceived stress was positively correlated with frequency of drinking to intoxication in the past month.

The purpose of the current study was to explore qualitatively the consequences of lesbians' bar attendance in a diverse urban setting. Parks (1999a) in one of the few studies that examined lesbian bars in depth, influenced the design of this study. She recruited participants from a rural community. They were all Caucasians, moderate to heavy drinkers, and had not previously been in treatment. That study found that participants' most consistent motivations for going to bars were to socialize, relax, have a good time with friends, be put at ease, and enhance conversation. Bar attendance increased when women were beginning to identify as a lesbian or were single, and older women were less likely to frequent the bars. Some women went to bars after games, especially when a bar sponsored their team.

## METHODS

### Sample

We recruited a total sample of 35 self-identified lesbians and bisexual women, using a snowball sampling technique, whereby we asked participants to recommend other women among their friends and colleagues as study participants. The participants had to be over the age of 21, female, and identify as either lesbian or bisexual. In addition, they had to be fluent in verbal and written English. They were not excluded based on their alcohol consumption or bar attendance. The eligibility criteria for the present study was different from those of Parks study in that we included women of color, women with disabilities, women in recovery, and women exhibiting varied drinking behavior. In addition, we recruited our study participants from the San Francisco Bay Area, an urban and politically liberal area. Parks subjects were from rural areas. Additionally, the data for this study were collected almost ten years after Parks' study.

We recruited initial participants via: the Internet; postings at San Francisco Bay Area LGBT community centers; and flyers posted and distributed at bars, restaurants, and other places frequented by lesbians. The participants were screened using a screening instrument over the telephone. We screened interested women and chose participants so as to have a racially and ethnically diverse sample, reflecting a range of alcohol consumption from abstinent to heavy drinkers. We used a matrix to try to recruit equal numbers of Caucasians, African Americans, Asian Americans and Latinas.

### Data Collection

The interview guide we developed was based on key concepts concerning lesbian health, stress, coping and substance use. The interviews were semi-structured. Specific questions relevant to this study included: Why are the bars important to you? Do the bars feel like a community for you? What do you do instead of frequenting the bars? Can you talk me through a negative experience in the bars? How about a positive experience? Do you ever drink to deal with stress? Do you go to the bars to deal with stress? What do you do outside of the bars to cope? The close-ended questions were followed up with open ended probes.

The first author (EG) conducted the interviews in private locations including respondents' homes, coffee shops, or the first author's office. Participants gave their written informed consent, and the Kaiser Permanente Institutional Review Board granted human subjects approval for the study protocol. The interviews averaged an hour in length, followed by a 10-15 minute written survey to collect demographic information and drinking history. Participants received a $20 gift certificate for their participation. We audio-taped and transcribed the interviews verbatim.

The first author took field notes directly following the interviews. These notes focused on observations about the interview, interviewer-participant rapport, participant nonverbal communication and demeanor, and any relevant methodological issues. We entered the field notes and the transcripts in Atlas.ti (1997), a software package for analyzing qualitative data.

## Data Analysis

Data analysis occurred iteratively as we proceeded with data collection. After several interviews were transcribed, we began coding the data. During this first phase of coding, the object was to capture the relevant aspects of the phenomena of interest and code with as much depth and breadth as possible without paying attention to the relative importance of the codes. These codes were reviewed in a graduate-level qualitative class at the University of California at San Francisco, several times. These codes were also examined by another author, Dr. Byrne, until Dr. Byrne and Dr. Gruskin reached agreement. Coding consistency was facilitated by using Atlas.ti which led us to build our list of codes.

The next step was to limit the data by making decisions about the relative salience of the codes. Here we identified the most frequently occurring codes. Responses occurring more or less frequently led us to find patterns in the data, which helped us to understand the role of the bar in lesbians' drinking behavior. We employed an explanatory matrix, a structure with which we organized codes into a logical configuration, to understand further relevant codes and how they were related. The parts of the explanatory matrix included: (1) the context in which the actions described by codes were embedded; (2) salient codes describing behaviors that facilitated, blocked, or shaped interactions; (3) codes describing processes or interactions that were caused by specific conditions; and (4) consequences or outcomes of specific processes or interactions. For the purposes of this paper, we focus on consequences.

Once we created the explanatory matrix, we conducted more interviews and asked participants specifically about the various aspects of the matrix, in an attempt to verify that it described the experiences of as many women as possible. We used these interviews to flesh out components of the developing conceptualizations that needed further support, elaboration, or clarification. The first author continued conducting 35 interviews until we reached theoretical saturation, a point at which codes were verified, and additional data revealed no new conceptual properties or dimensions (Glaser & Strauss 1967; Strauss 1987).

To have further conceptual and methodological verification, we presented the results of our study to a doctoral level medical sociology and nursing class, a psychologist, a psychiatrist, several colleagues at the

Division of Research at Kaiser Permanente, and other lay people, both lesbians and heterosexuals. We also received feedback when the paper was presented at a professional conference.

## FINDINGS

### Sociodemographics and Alcohol Use

Study participants were highly educated and diverse in both race/ethnicity and age (see Table 1). All except five of the women had gone to a bar in the last month or two leading up to their interview for this study. Most of the women were connected to the lesbian community, indicating that they participated in activities in the lesbian, gay, bisexual and, transgender community through online chats, use of websites, volunteering, religious groups, twelve step programs, other self help groups, sports events, political events, pride events, bookstores, bars and reading lesbian newspapers or magazines. Three of the women reported zero to three of the above activities, sixteen of the women reported four to six activities, and sixteen reported seven or more activities.

A fairly wide range of alcohol consumption was reported among participants. Ten women drank one drink or less per week, eighteen women drank between 1.25 and 3.5 drinks per week, and seven women drank six or more drinks per week. The way that the question was set up, we classified the women either less than 3.5 drinks or over 6.0 drinks, which unfortunately left an unassessed gap of 3.5-6 drinks per week. Twenty-two women were concerned about their alcohol use at some point in their lives, whereas only three women were still concerned about their alcohol use at the time of the survey.

We present the four main dimensions of the explanatory matrix that provide a structure for understanding the consequences of participants' bar attendance: safety and support across the life course; lesbian identity development; reduction of stress; and social networks and intimate relationships.

### Safety and Support Over the Life Course

Overwhelmingly, participants reported feeling more comfortable when in lesbian bars than when in primarily heterosexual bars, both because discrimination was less likely in this environment and because bars were perceived by participants as safe places:

TABLE 1. Characteristics of study participants (N = 35)

| Age (range 22-55 years) | N | % |
|---|---|---|
| 20-29 years | 10 | 29% |
| 30-39 years | 12 | 32% |
| 40-49 years | 9 | 26% |
| 50-55 years | 4 | 12% |
| | | |
| **Race/ethnicity (self identified)** | | |
| White | 16 | 47% |
| Black | 2 | 6% |
| Asian | 6 | 15% |
| Latina | 3 | 9% |
| Native American | 1 | 3% |
| Jewish | 2 | 6% |
| Indian | 1 | 3% |
| Multi-racial | 4 | 12% |
| | | |
| **Education** | | |
| High School Graduate | 2 | 6% |
| Some College | 4 | 8% |
| College Graduate | 18 | 52% |
| Graduate School | 10 | 29% |
| Unknown | 1 | 3% |

*Irene, 41 years*

I don't know why community was important . . . who was I as a lesbian? They didn't assume anything about you in particular . . . That was where you could not have to have a barrier around you.

Participants also described the bars as a place to find their culture and chosen family:

*Lisa, 35 years*

I have no idea why we ended up there (after the announcement that gay marriages would be performed in San Francisco). For me personally, it's about either celebrating or supporting each other. And that's one of the reasons why I go (to the bars). So the importance for me is mostly the support network. I don't know what other people's intentions are. I just go for the community.

This need for community and family was especially important for participants because they often felt stress in other communities and relationships when their sexual orientation was not accepted. Because they were born into families consisting mostly of heterosexuals, lesbians in this study often reported not having the immediate and unconditional support of their families and communities of origin, especially when they first disclosed their sexual orientation to their families.

The need for support and community was especially evident in interviews with participants of color. These women suggested that the stress of being a double minority caused them to seek bars specifically catering to lesbians of color to minimize the discrimination that they encountered based on their race/ethnicity in other lesbian spaces and in heterosexual bars:

*May, early 30s*

Yeah, I think that definitely there's that pressure because for some reason there's still that division between different ethnic groups in the lesbian community . . . I've been to events where [it's] predominantly lesbians of color, [and] the atmosphere is different. It's much more relaxing and we feel like we can accept each other. I mean, we can be ourselves, basically, and it's a struggle for me because I don't want to be like that. I want people to just see me who I am and don't judge me.

Large women experienced stress related to size discrimination, in addition to that experienced as a result of being lesbian and/or women of color:

*Jane, 37 years*

So, you know, in the lesbian community and being gay and being a person of color, being a big person, you know, it's all those stresses. They take a toll on you. And sometimes you just don't want to feel it. You just want to, like, be out and have fun. And sometimes you need alcohol or drugs or whatever, because then you don't feel so self-conscious about being who you are. And that's sad . . .

Minority participants described choosing bars catering to lesbians of color to combat the discrimination they experienced within Caucasian-dominated lesbian bars, suggesting that Caucasian lesbian patrons reproduced patterns of racial discrimination found in the United States.

## Lesbian Identity Development

Community connection fostered by bar attendance was an important part of participants' lesbian identity development, both in terms of "coming out" and learning about sexual behavior.

### Monique, 39 years

I did some of my coming out in gay bars. And what I really loved ... was that sense of community and like . . . a sense of family . . .

Other participants discussed the early phases of coming out before feeling fully comfortable with their sexual orientation. In this stage, they would seek approval and understanding from other lesbians, women whom they could easily locate in the bars. Participants described experimenting with flirting and with sexuality that was sometimes made easier with alcohol. Other participants emphasized the importance of the bar to young women, although lesbian bars were also important for older women for some of the same reasons.

## Reduction of Stress

While lesbian bars are unique drinking establishments with regard to lesbian identity development, safety and support, they are similar to mainstream bars in many ways. Our participants reported, at one time or another, going to the bar to "blow off steam" and drink alcohol.

### Joanne, 27 years

Sometimes I drink because of family things or just feeling stressed out about life in general. Just work is–I have pressure from work and I have . . . I don't know, maybe problems with friends or things that I can't deal with.

Using alcohol to cope with stress became dangerous when not consumed in moderation.

*Beth, 47 years*

> Once in a while, when I'm in a situation where I feel that I don't
> have a lot of control, then I get really, really drunk to forget, be-
> cause . . . it's like a shield for me. Then my sensory mode is really
> low and I don't have to feel anything. I can be numb, you know.

Several of the participants also were coping with chronic physical or
psychological illnesses. They reported drinking to self-medicate and
deal with stress.

*Maggie, 37 years*

> I have trouble with depression, and it was a self-medication thing
> [drinking to excess]. And it was very much a coping-with-stress
> mechanism. I was, I guess, a binge drinker. And it was very much
> self-medication for depression.

### Social Networks and Intimate Relationships

Along with meeting women with whom to have friendships, lesbians
found sexual and intimate partners in the bars. Participants related that it
was difficult to find places for recreation that were accepting of lesbian
sexual orientation, and this need drew lesbians into the bars.

Lesbians' relationship status often determined the role that the bar
played in their lives. The perceived lack of places to find lesbians with
whom to have relationships led lesbians to the bars where they knew
that single women were available. Some participants spoke of a sense of
desperation they observed in some women who had not had luck finding partners in other places:

*Jane, 37 years*

> As [women] get older, they want to have a partner, want to have a
> house . . . want to share their lives together, want to settle down.
> And [they're not finding] that in the bar, but I think that a lot of
> women feel desperate to go, to have this partner, too, you know?
> So where are you going to find women? In the bar.

Women often reported that they would leave the bar scene when they
had partners, and then come back again when they broke up and were
ready to start dating. However, participants also reported that if they

were partnered with women who went to the bars regularly, they might have continued to frequent the bars:

*Sue, 38 years*

> When I was in college, yes [I went to the bars more frequently]. And, in spaces in my life when I've been single, I drank more. I was with a woman for ten years who didn't drink. Not that she didn't want me to drink, but it didn't lend itself to situations where . . . . I mean we would go out and stuff, but more than not, I was at home, nesting.

When women formed relationships with non-drinking women, they tended to reduce their drinking. Either way, partners had an influence on some women's bar attendance.

*Jane, 37 years*

> I think for the young dykes, alcohol is great. And alcohol encompasses their sexuality. You go out to drink; it means you get loose. If you get loose, then you want to party . . . Lesbians need to feel sexual. Lesbians are very desexualized by this culture . . . Alcohol helps us to be sexual. So alcohol is perceived as a sexy thing, like drugs, as opposed to a writing group. [Laughs] . . . "We want to go to the bar! That's where the sex is!"

While using alcohol to reduce inhibitions made meeting people easier, it also led to negative behaviors such as drug use or unsafe sex, according to many participants. All pointed to the link between socializing at the bar and using alcohol while there.

It is important to note that the bar community was not seen as positive by all.

*Joanne, 27 years*

> . . . Even though it's in a superficial environment it's like well, at least you're not by yourself then I can forget whatever difficulties I'm having.

Another participant explained that non-drinkers could be pressured to imbibe even if one did not have the express intention to drink while at the bar:

*Jane, 37 years*

> But you almost feel, like, obligated to drink. "Well, wow, what are you drinking?" "I'm not drinking anything." "What?! Why?!" "Uh, I'll have a drink of water." "You can't drink water!" "Well, yeah, I can. Watch me," you know? It's like there's this pressure to drink when you go in the bar too. So it's not like you can just go to the bar and just hang out. I mean, you could, but people want you to drink because they're drinking, and they want you to have the same reality that they're having, which is a drunk one . . .

While participants sought and often found friends and romantic partners in the lesbian bars, they described situations when excessive drinking in bars resulted in stress on women's relationships including those with intimate partners:

*Beth, 47 years*

> One of my earlier girlfriends was an alcoholic and drug addict. It's kind of making me so uncomfortable where people pay a lot of money for alcohol and they just drink one after another until they are really, really drunk; really, really wasted. It wasn't very much fun for me anymore.

This drinking occurred in tandem with increased tobacco and illicit drug use.

*Josie, 31 years*

> Oh, God! That was the worst part [heavy drinking, heavy bar use] So you still have all the alcohol stuff on top of, you know, your credit being ruined, losing jobs, not having a driver's license, burning all kinds of bridges, your family not talking to you–plus the fact that you're stoned, you're fucking God knows what, and you feel disgusted about yourself. And who you are and not being able to numb the pain.

## DISCUSSION

As previously stated, the purpose of the current study was to explore qualitatively the consequences of lesbians' bar attendance in a diverse urban setting. The findings suggest, that seeking to understand better the consequences of frequenting the lesbian bar is a deceivingly complex problem. As identified in the literature (Bloomfield, 1993; Heffernan, 1998; Parks 1999a), we found that lesbians still frequent bars. In our discussion of the findings, we focus on the inevitable health tradeoffs made by participants when frequenting the lesbian bar, the psychosocial importance of the bar to participants in this study, and the connection between minority stress and alcohol use. Within these sections, we also discuss implications of our findings for public health interventions. Finally, we identify the limitations of this study.

### Health Tradeoffs

Whenever we attempted to describe the types of positive outcomes found in our study and in Parks' study such as finding an extended community, feeling safety, developing sexual identity, and social recreation, we realized that attendant negative outcomes also occurred. For example, while Jane found safety in being out in the lesbian bar ("You just want to be out and have fun"), she used drugs to deal with her self-conscious feelings ("And sometimes you need alcohol and drugs or whatever") and felt pressure from bar patrons and bartenders to use alcohol. The inverse was also true: when we explored what seemed at first to be purely negative results of frequenting the lesbian bar–such as the binge drinking described by Maggie to self-medicate her depression and stress–we could not ignore the positive influence on participants of being among the bar patrons in what was perceived as a community setting, such as when Lisa explained that "the importance for me is mostly the support network."

These findings suggest that public health interventions in this context should be guided by a philosophy of harm reduction. A harm reduction approach in this context concedes that alcohol is the "lure" of the lesbian bar and strives for ways to minimize the negative consequences of alcohol abuse while retaining the positive consequences of the bar for its patrons. One intervention that builds upon a harm reduction approach would be for health educators and providers to work with bar owners to educate them about alcohol abuse in the lesbian community and to develop strategies to minimize this problem among bar patrons.

Another, more radical, intervention is to "redefine" the lesbian bar. In other words, we suggest developing and marketing social spaces and events that both retain the festive and sexy atmosphere of the lesbian bar, as well as meet bar patrons' social, psychological, and cultural needs, but emphasize moderate or no use of alcohol. While this solution might not attract those bar patrons who seek out the lesbian bar to get drunk, get numb, self-medicate, or otherwise abuse alcohol, it could provide a solution for those bar patrons who are looking for ways to avoid compromising their health in the pursuit of community, romance, support, or identity.

### Psychosocial Importance of the Lesbian Bar

In the previous discussion of tradeoffs, Lisa and Jane were cited as examples of participants who received positive consequences by frequenting lesbian bars. Examining their words more deeply reveals that neither participant sought the bar itself–the physical location or the alcohol available there–instead, they went to interact with the other lesbians who were at the bar. In other words, these participants were fulfilling psychosocial needs by going to the bar. When a participant went to the lesbian bar for a "support network" or so that a participant could "be out," she was using the bar to reduce stress, find safety and support, enhance lesbian identity development, and build social networks. The physical location of the bar itself became a culturally agreed upon "staging area" for the fulfillment of social and psychological needs.

The results of this study build upon Parks'(1999a) study, even though Parks gathered her data over ten years ago in another part of the country and without as diverse a sample. Both Parks' study and the present study found the following positive consequences to bar attendance: participants met other women for friends and dating; they tended to frequent the bars when they were young and single; they often adjusted their drinking patterns to match those of their partners; their drinking increased when they started or ended relationships; they went to the bar to relax and cope with stress; and they used the bars to deal with depression, anger, and anxiety. Also similar to the current study, most of the women in Parks' study reported negative consequences from drinking. This included physical health effects, legal consequences, work impairment, and behavior incongruent with their image of themselves or their values.

Findings from the present study move beyond Parks, however. This study identifies the complex mix of positive and negative consequences of bar patronage. It also connects bar patronage to larger psychosocial needs of bar patrons, such as the importance of the bar scene to women who are in the early stages of lesbian identity development and seek social networks. Finally, the present study focuses on implications for public health interventions.

If health providers and educators could be assisted in understanding the psychosocial importance of the bar scene in lesbians' lives, they would be better positioned to promote positive behavior within the lesbian community. To help the lesbian who has problems with alcohol to seek positive sources of support, health care providers and health educators should realize the role that the bar and other drinking venues are playing in this problem. For example, Sue explained that "in spaces in my life when I've been single, I drank more." For Sue, increased alcohol use was intertwined with her periodic seeking of romantic partners. Suggesting that the lesbian remove herself from the bar scene is asking her to give up a social space that validates, entertains, relaxes and provides partners and community. Working with their lesbian clients to limit their drinking in the bars and to find other places to meet these needs may be helpful.

## *Minority Stress and Alcohol Use*

One way for health educators and providers to understand better the connection between the lesbian bar and alcohol use is to frame bar patron alcohol abuse in terms of minority stress. Researchers have found that minority stress–the perceived pressure of negative life events and associated stigma resulting from discrimination based on race, ethnicity, gender, and/or sexual orientation–is a fact of life for lesbians and bisexual women. The findings from this study show that some lesbians cope with this stress by frequenting lesbian bars. Heffernan (1998) and Beatty et al. (1999) found that stress was higher for lesbians than for the general population of women. Specifically, lesbians may have high levels of stress due to their inability to accept their lesbian identity (VanScoy, 1997), isolation (VanScoy, 1997), difficulties in managing self-disclosure at work (Hughes & Wilsnack, 1997; Nawyn et al., 2000), the stressors of coping with non-supportive families of origin (Beatty et al., 1999; Hughes & Wilsnack, 1997) and experiences of discrimination. Most participants in this study reported seeking the lesbian bar to be comfortably out and avoid discrimination because of their sexual orientation.

Further, when a participant used drugs and alcohol "to deal with self-conscious feelings" about being lesbian while she was in the lesbian bar, this suggests that she has internalized negative societal attitudes (Meyer, 2003) which leads to alcohol abuse. In addition, when a participant sought out the lesbian bar so that she could "be out," she demonstrated an expectation of stressful events related to her sexual orientation (Meyer, 2003). If health care providers or educators are able to understand the link between alcohol abuse and the high level of stress caused by discrimination/marginalization in society, they may be able better to design interventions within the psychosocial context of the lesbian bar.

## Limitations

A major limitation of this study was the high educational level of most of the participants, which limits the generalizability of the findings. It is unclear whether lesbians have a higher level of education than heterosexuals, or if it is a sampling or participation bias, or a combination of both. In addition, because of the methods used for recruitment, we were not able to compute eligibility and participation rates and thus cannot directly assess representativeness and potential for participation bias. Future quantitative research, which could test the premise presented in this paper, could also address this sampling issue.

The generalizability of the findings were also limited by the geographic context of the sample. This study included women who lived in the San Francisco Bay Area with its large and visible lesbian population. In addition, almost all of the women who participated in this study were connected to the lesbian community in some way. Finally, the questions in the survey were created for this study and not from validated scales. Thus the accuracy and precision of the measures studied are not known.

## POLICY IMPLICATIONS

It was surprising that many women did not know about non-drinking community alternatives to the bar, such as book readings or performance art. To publicize such options, we suggest a public health social marketing campaign that would highlight alternatives to bars. Though it is unlikely that non-drinking establishments will completely replace lesbian bars, it is important for health educators and providers to work with bar owners to conduct education on alcohol abuse. It also might be feasible to encourage bars to serve a wider variety of non-alcoholic drinks in an economically viable way so that their business is not solely dependent on the amount of alcoholic drinks purchased. Health professionals could encourage bar owners to host entertainment where the focus is not on drinking. The receptivity of bar owners to these interventions is one area for future research. Also, quantitative studies can determine the generalizability of this study to the general population or lesbians and bisexual women.

## REFERENCES

Aaron, D. J., Markovic, N., Danielson, M. E., Honnold, J. A., Janosky, J. E., & Schmidt, N. J. (2001). Behavioral risk factors for disease and preventive health practices among lesbians. *Am J Public Health, 91*(6), 972-975.

Beatty, R., Geckle, M., Huggins, J., Kapner, C., Lewis, K., & Sanstrom, D. (1999). Gay men, lesbians and bisexuals. In B. McCrady & E. Epstein (Eds.), *Addictions: A comprehensive guide book* (pp. 542-551). New York: Oxford University Press.

Bergmark, K. H. (1999). Drinking in the swedish gay and lesbian community. *Drug Alcohol Depend, 56*(2), 133-143.

Bloomfield, K. (1993). A comparison of alcohol consumption between lesbians and heterosexual women in an urban population. *Drug Alcohol Depend, 33*(3), 257-269.

Cochran, S. D., Keenan, C., Schober, C., & Mays, V. M. (2000). Estimates of alcohol use and clinical treatment needs among homosexually active men and women in the U.S. population. *J Consult Clin Psychol, 68*(6), 1062-1071.

Diamant, A. L., Wold, C., Spritzer, K., & Gelberg, L. (2000). Health behaviors, health status, and access to and use of health care: A population-based study of lesbian, bisexual, and heterosexual women. *Arch Fam Med, 9*(10), 1043-1051.

Dibble, S. L., Roberts, S. A., & Nussey, B. (2004). Comparing breast cancer risk between lesbians and their heterosexual sisters. *Womens Health Issues, 14*(2), 60-68.

Drabble, L., Midanik, L., & Trocki, K. (2005). Reports of alcohol consumption and alcohol related problems among homosexual, bisexual and heterosexual respondents: Results from the 2000 national alcohol survey.

Faderman, L. (1991). *Odd girls and twilight lovers.* New York: Columbia University Press.

Gilman, S. E., Cochran, S. D., Mays, V. M., Hughes, M., Ostrow, D., & Kessler, R. C. (2001). Risk of psychiatric disorders among individuals reporting same-sex sexual partners in the national comorbidity survey. *Am J Public Health, 91*(6), 933-939.

Gruskin, E. P., Hart, S., Gordon, N., & Ackerson, L. (2001). Patterns of cigarette smoking and alcohol use among lesbians and bisexual women enrolled in a large health maintenance organization. *Am J Public Health, 91*(6), 976-979.

Heffernan, K. (1998). The nature and predictors of substance use among lesbians. *Addict Behav, 23*(4), 517-528.

Hughes, T. L. (2003). Lesbians' drinking patterns: Beyond the data. *Subst Use Misuse, 38*(11-13), 1739-1758.

Hughes, T. L., & Wilsnack, S. C. (1997). Use of alcohol among lesbians: Research and clinical implications. *Am J Orthopsychiatry, 67*(1), 20-36.

Mays, V. M., Yancey, A. K., Cochran, S. D., Weber, M., & Fielding, J. E. (2002). Heterogeneity of health disparities among african american, hispanic, and asian american women: Unrecognized influences of sexual orientation. *Am J Public Health,* *92*(4), 632-639.

Meyer, I. H. (2003). Prejudice, social stress, and mental health in lesbian, gay, and bisexual populations: Conceptual issues and research evidence. *Psychol Bull, 129*(5), 674-697.

Nawyn, S. J., Richman, J. A., Rospenda, K. M., & Hughes, T. L. (2000). Sexual identity and alcohol-related outcomes: Contributions of workplace harassment. *J Subst Abuse, 11*(3), 289-304.

Parks, C. (1999a). Lesbians social drinking: The role of alcohol in growing up and living as lesbian. *Contemporary Drug Problems, 26*(Spring), 75-129.

Parks, C. A. (1999b). Lesbian identity development: An examination of differences across generations. *Am J Orthopsychiatry, 69*(3), 347-361.

Sandfort, T. G., de Graaf, R., Bijl, R. V., & Schnabel, P. (2001). Same-sex sexual behavior and psychiatric disorders: Findings from the netherlands mental health survey and incidence study (nemesis). *Arch Gen Psychiatry, 58*(1), 85-91.

Skinner, W. F., & Otis, M. D. (1996). Drug and alcohol use among lesbian and gay people in a southern U.S. sample: Epidemiological, comparative, and methodological findings from the trilogy project. *J Homosex, 30*(3), 59-92.

VanScoy, H. (1997). Health behaviors in lesbians. In D. Gochman (Ed.), *Handbook of health behavior research iii: Demography, development and diversity* (pp. 141-160). New York: Plenum Press.

Wolfe, M. (1997). Invisible women in invisible places. In G. Ingram, A. Bouthillette & Y. Retter (Eds.), *Queers in space* (pp. 301-324). Seattle: Bay Press.

doi:10.1300/J013v44n02_06

# Comparing Sexual Minority Status Across Sampling Methods and Populations

Deborah J. Bowen, PhD
Judith Bradford, PhD
Diane Powers, MA

**SUMMARY.** The health of sexual minority women (SMW) has recently received research attention. Previous research into the health of SMW (e.g., lesbians, bisexuals, transgendered women) used a mixture of sampling methods, many of which were poorly documented and difficult to understand. The results of these previous studies do not present a consistent pattern of findings, possibly due to differences in sampling methods. The present study compared the characteristics of SMW across four survey sampling methods, three in the same geographic area. Differences were found among groups of SMW by sampling method, including in demographic data (e.g., level of education) and personal

Deborah J. Bowen is affiliated with the Cancer Prevention Program, Fred Hutchinson Cancer Research Cancer and Health Services, University of Washington.

Judith Bradford is affiliated with Virginia Commonwealth University and Fenway Community Health Center.

Diane Powers is affiliated with the Psychiatry & Behavioral Sciences, University of Washington.

Address correspondence to: Deborah J. Bowen, PhD, Fred Hutchinson Cancer Research Center, 1100 Fairview Avenue N, M3-B232, Seattle, WA 98109 (E-mail: dbowen@fhcrc.org).

This research was funded by grants from the National Human Genome Research Institute (HG01190) and the National Cancer Institute (CA79654).

[Haworth co-indexing entry note]: "Comparing Sexual Minority Status Across Sampling Methods and Populations." Bowen, Deborah J., Judith Bradford, and Diane Powers. Co-published simultaneously in *Women & Health* (The Haworth Medical Press, an imprint of The Haworth Press, Inc.) Vol. 44, No. 2, 2006, pp. 121-134; and: *Preventive Health Measures for Lesbian and Bisexual Women* (ed: Shelly Kerr, and Robin Mathy) The Haworth Medical Press, an imprint of The Haworth Press, Inc., 2006, pp. 121-134. Single or multiple copies of this article are available for a fee from The Haworth Document Delivery Service [1-800-HAWORTH, 9:00 a.m. - 5:00 p.m. (EST). E-mail address: docdelivery@haworthpress.com].

health data (e.g., rates of regular mammography screening). These findings provided a possible explanation for the variety of findings in the published literature and identified rigorous sampling methods that can be used in future research. doi:10.1300/J013v44n02_07 *[Article copies available for a fee from The Haworth Document Delivery Service: 1-800-HAWORTH. E-mail address: <docdelivery@haworthpress.com> Website: <http://www. HaworthPress.com> © 2006 by The Haworth Press, Inc. All rights reserved.]*

**KEYWORDS.** Sexual minority women, obesity, intervention design, focus groups

Sexual minority women, or women who define themselves as lesbian, bisexual, gay, or transgendered, may be at higher risk for poorer health outcomes than heterosexual women (Committee on Lesbian Health Research Priorities, 1999). Sexual minority women (SMW) may face higher health risks as compared to heterosexual women because of differential rates of health behaviors (Bradford et al., 1994; Burnett et al., 1999; Deevy, 1990; Polena et al., 1994; Powers et al., 2001; Roberts & Sorensen, 1999; Trippet & Bain, 1992; Valanis et al., 2000; White & Dull, 1997) and because of economic and socio-cultural barriers to appropriate health care (Bradford et al., 1994; Bybee & Roeder, 1990; Susan D. Cochran & Mays, 1988; Lehmann et al., 1998; Mathews et al., 1986; Randall, 1989; Stevens & Hall, 1988; Warchafsky, 1992); however, variability in data reported in the literature makes the existing published literature difficult to interpret. For example, a recent review of tobacco use rates among lesbians and gay men under consideration for publication concluded that it is likely that sexual minority individuals use tobacco at a higher rate than the general population, but the diversity of rates reported in the literature (from 8% to 70%) makes this conclusion uncertain (Ryan et al., 2001). Similarly, rates of mammography screening among SMW vary across studies, from 40% to 70% (Bradford et al., 1994; Valanis et al., 2000), with estimates from larger samples and more generalizable samples somewhat lower than from non-probability samples, making conclusions regarding breast cancer risk and diagnosis difficult. However, very few probability samples of SMW have been drawn, due to lack of research funding and relative rarity in the general population.

One possible explanation for this variability in health behavior rates is the quality of the sampling in currently published articles. We know very little about the actual population rates of such health related issues because of the use of non-population based sampling methods (Ganguli et al., 1998; Kish, 1965; Meyer & Colten, 1999; Sell & Petrulio, 1996). Many of the early studies of the health and health habits of SMW were conducted in volunteer samples (Bradford et al., 1994), providing little ability to generalize to any sort of larger population. Later studies were conducted as part of a randomized clinical trial (Valanis et al., 2000). The sampling method in the latter study was still not population-based so generalizability will be low. Some recent studies (S. D. Cochran & Mays, 2000; Diamant et al., 2000) (D. J. Bowen et al., 2004; Stall et al., 2003) have used rigorous population-based sampling methods, but there have been no direct comparisons of their sampling methods and their data. Researchers do not understand the relationship between sampling method and information collected from women of differing sexual orientations, and this important step must be taken before we can make any judgments regarding true estimates of the health behavior rates for SMW.

We present here the results of four surveys that we have conducted within a two-year time period measuring sexual orientation using different sampling methods. The first three were conducted in the same geographical area. The fourth study, though conducted in a different city, provides a comparison with area probability sampling. For each, we present the yield of SMW, our judgments about the generalizability of the sample, and information on health behavior rates. The aim of this paper is to compare the participant data and demographic and health-related data among the four surveys. Examining these methodologies will allow us to re-interpret some of the confusing data from previous studies on SMW and to design better sampling methods for the future. We hypothesized that samples recruited using volunteer non-probability methods would report more health-oriented behaviors, such as screening and nonsmoking status.

## *METHOD*

### *Study A–Volunteer Sample of Women*

*Sampling.* Eligibility requirements included being a woman aged 18-74 years, living within 60 miles of the research center in Seattle, Washington, and willingness to complete the study requirements of randomization to intervention or control and longitudinal follow up. Methodological details are presented elsewhere (Deborah J. Bowen et al.,

2002). Notices were placed in newspapers and local health-related centers asking for women interested in learning more about their breast cancer risk to call a number and leave contact information. All calls were returned for a discussion of possible study participation, which involved survey completion and randomization into either a counseling intervention of breast cancer risk counseling or a control group for an ongoing study.

*Survey Methods.* Interested participants were sent a written self-administered questionnaire and a preaddressed envelope for return. If participants did not return the questionnaire within two weeks, they received a telephone call to remind them to complete the survey. Two months later the acceptance window for each participant closed.

## Study B–Volunteer Sample of Sexual Minority Women

*Sampling.* The eligibility criteria for this study were identical to the previous one, with the addition that all participants self-identify as SMW (e.g., lesbian, bisexual, gay, queer). Notices were placed in newspapers and community resources for the SMW community inviting women to call and leave their contact information if they were interested in learning more about breast cancer risk.

*Survey Methods.* Interested participants were sent a self-administered questionnaire and a preaddressed envelope for return. If participants did not return the questionnaire within two weeks, they received a telephone call to remind them to complete the survey. Two months later the acceptance window for each participant closed.

## Study C–Population Based Telephone Survey of Women

*Sampling.* Eligible participants for this project were women who were between 18 and 74 years old, lived within 60 miles of the research center in Seattle, WA, had not been previously diagnosed with breast cancer, had a working telephone number and address, spoke English, planned to be in their present residence for at least one year, and were willing to complete the survey requirements of randomization to intervention or control and longitudinal follow up. The investigators purchased names from Mailing Lists Plus, a company that brokers name lists for research projects. Mailing Lists Plus obtained lists and the contact information by using both public (voter registration and driver's license rolls) and private sources (credit bureaus, insurance lists, and other lists of names) with coverage claims of between 85% and 90% of adult residents in the geographic area. Study staff mailed a consent letter to randomly selected persons on the list fitting the age and gender criteria of our study. We followed all mailings with telephone contact to determine eligibility and interest and to conduct the survey.

*Survey Methods.* Trained interviewers contacted each sampled person by telephone to complete a 15-minute screening survey by telephone. If eligible and interested, participants then completed the baseline survey by telephone. Interviewers made up to 15 attempts at varied times of day to contact participants who had received the consent letter. Each participant's data was collected or not during a 2-month window.

## Study D–Area Probability Sample of Women

*Sampling.* Census (2000) data were used to identify "lesbian couple-rich" census tracts in Boston, MA, meaning that 0.75% of the households were female-partnered. Boston was selected as the site for this study because of the availability of a co-investigator (JB) and interviewers. For each census tract, we counted the percent of households with a female head of household and a second female identified as "unmarried partner." Using Atlas Global Information Systems software, a map of the Boston area was prepared showing zip code and census tract boundaries. We selected Jamaica Plain (zip 02130) as the target zip code.

*Survey Methods.* Eligibility criteria for this study include being female, living in a residence within our defined geographic area, aged 18 years and older, and being able to complete in-person interview or self-administered survey in English (D. J. Bowen et al., 2004). Interviewers approached and screened randomly selected households within segments. Interviewers approached a sampled household and attempted to complete the screening survey to determine eligibility with the first adult household member they personally encountered at the door. The data were conducted using a "choice" method: at the time of request, each sampled person chose whether to complete the self-administered questionnaire with the interviewer present or mail the self-completed questionnaire back later. If there was more than one eligible household member, the sampled person was randomly selected from among the eligible persons. The data were collected over 6 months.

## Common Measures

In all four studies we identified a core set of common questionnaire items to present comparable data. We collected demographic information using the same simple, single-item measures in each study (What was the highest level of education you obtained? Are you married, single, divorced, separated, or living with a partner? What is your race or ethnic status? How old are you?). Perceived breast cancer risk was assessed using the same single item measure in which participants rated their chances of ever getting breast cancer on a continuous scale of 0 to 100 (Weinstein & Klein, 1995). Mammography screening was assessed using two questions (When was your last mammogram? When was the one before the last one?), which are based on the definition of regular mammography: obtaining at least two mammograms in the past three years (Urban et al., 1995). Data for this question is presented only for women aged 40 years and older due to the relevance of mammography for the older age group. Intentions to obtain mammography screening that matched age-appropriate recommendations were measured by asking women if they intended to obtain screening on a 4-point scale with anchors of "strongly disagree" to "strongly agree" (Andersen & Urban, 1997). Smoking status from the CDC's Behavioral Risk Factor Survey (current smoker now) was also collected in the same manner in each of the four studies. Mental health was measured using a subscale of the SF-36 Health Survey for Perceived Quality of Life, a well validated, reliable, and widely used instrument that includes 36 items (Hays & Morales, 2001). This self-report scale measures the following eight health concepts: physical functioning, role-physical, role-emotional, bodily pain, general health, vitality, social functioning, mental health, and reported health transition.

We measured sexual orientation in all studies using a similar (but not identical) question that asked participants to mark the category that best applied to them: lesbian, gay, homosexual, bisexual, heterosexual, transgendered, or other (with fill-in option). For all studies, we collapsed the sexual minority categories (i.e., not heterosexual) to calculate the proportion of the sample that were sexual minority women. The "other" category was reviewed in all studies and was collapsed into either heterosexual or SMW.

## Analyses

First we considered the properties of each recruitment method and made judgments about relevant properties (e.g., generalizability) of each. Next we compared the recruitment patterns of SMW for the four studies by comparing the recruitment yields across the studies. We compared data from the surveys using analysis of variance (with Tukey's test for pair-wise comparisons) for continuous data and chi-square tests for categorical data. According to the method of Sudman (1983), each sample can be assigned a generalizability score, from $-5$ to 20 (higher is better), and samples' scores can be compared to obtain a sense of sample quality. Elements considered in this generalizability score include the geographic spread of each sample, acknowledgment of study limitations, and use of special populations. Based on this scale, we assigned each sample a generalizability score.

## RESULTS

Table 1 shows the recruitment process data for the four survey samples. All yields were calculated as overall response rates for the entire sample using the principles of the American Association of Public Opinion Research, Method #4 (American Association for Public Opinion Research web site, 2003). In addition to yields, we provided information about the characteristics of the sample, including the proportion of the sample that self-labeled as SMW, the comparability to a similarly recruited heterosexual sample, and the cost of the sample per recruited participant. Table 1 presents judgments about the quality of the sampling method (Sudman, 1983) based on the extent to which the sample

TABLE 1. Recruitment for sexual minority status in four surveys of women.

| | Study A | Study B | Study C | Study D |
|---|---|---|---|---|
| | Volunteer sample of women | Volunteer sample of sexual minority women | Population-based telephone survey | Area probability household survey |
| Number of initial contacts/attempts | 799 | 206 | 4608 | 737 |
| Number (%) eligible | 518 (64%) | 192 (93%) | 1934 (42%) | 335 (45%) |
| Response number and yield (%) | 357 (69%) | 150 (78%) | 1366 (70%) | 208 (62%) |
| % SMW | 4% | 100% | 5% | 16% |
| Generalizability Score | 0 | 0 | 5 | 5 |
| Comparability to Heterosexual sample | Low | Low to medium | Medium | High |
| Cost | Low | Low | Medium | High |

was likely to represent the population. Scores varied across samples, from relatively low scores for the volunteer non-probability samples (A and B) to higher scores for the quality of probability sample in Study C and Study D. The methods used in these latter studies were specifically selected to allow for generalizing to a population. Given the reasonable response rates in the population-based studies, it is acceptable to generalize to a population from these samples (Studies C and D).

As seen in this table, response rates varied only slightly across the sampling methods, from 60% to 75%. The yield of SMW was high in Study B due to the targeted recruitment messages and strategies. The yield of SMW women was different in Study D compared to the others, possibly due to conducting the study in a geographic region that was selected because census data indicated it contained a relatively high level of same sex partnered households. The comparability of the SMW sample to a heterosexual sample (e.g., the examples of A, C, or D) was judged to be variable, depending on method of recruitment used. The willingness of women to report their sexual orientation may vary between Studies A and B resulting in different reporting biases. The comparability of the SMW in Studies C and D was judged as higher because recruitment in these two studies was proactive and did not depend on women feeling comfortable responding to an advertisement for a research project on breast cancer risk education; however, there might be differences between Studies C and D in reporting sexual orientation because of the demands of face-to-face reporting.

We estimated the cost to recruit participants for each study, by estimating the total number of hours spent on recruiting participants. We did not have cost data to compare costs quantitatively across the projects. Costs differed across the studies, with volunteer samples (A and B) representing the least expensive methods of recruitment (participants volunteer for entry into these studies) and area probability sampling (D) the most expensive (interviewers visit households and actively solicit participation from eligible residents).

Table 2 shows the demographic data for SMW across the four samples. These data varied across the studies, providing support for the idea that the samples differ in their ability to inform about the population. The area probability sample had significantly lower percentages of women with college education and women in current partnership with another woman than did the other three samples.

Comparisons of health-related variables between SMW in the four samples are presented in Table 3. We found differences in some of these variables across the four sampling methods. The proportion of women

TABLE 2. Demographic comparisons for sexual minority women across four surveys.

| | Study A | Study B | Study C | Study D |
|---|---|---|---|---|
| | Volunteer sample of women | Volunteer sample of sexual minority women | Population-based telephone survey | Area probability household survey[a] |
| Age ($\overline{X}$, SD) | 46 (12) | 44 (12) | 40 (11) | 37.1(11) |
| % Caucasian | 93% | 90% | 92% | 80% |
| % with post-college experience* | 75% | 86% | 65% | 47% |
| % partnered* | 73% | 70% | 65% | 53% |

*Significant differences among studies; $p < 0.05$
[a] These analyses were weighted for clustering of households from the original sample.

TABLE 3. Comparisons of health-related variables in sexual minority women across four surveys.

| | Study A | Study B | Study C | Study D |
|---|---|---|---|---|
| | Volunteer sample of women | Volunteer sample of sexual minority women | Population-based telephone survey | Area probability household survey[a] |
| Regular mammography screener?* | 76% | 62% | 51% | 45% |
| Current smoker? | 8% | 7% | 12% | 17% |
| Perceived risk of breast cancer* $\overline{X}$ (SD), range = 0-100% | 56% (6) | 64% (8) | 54% (7) | 43% (8) |
| Mental Health* $\overline{X}$ (SD), range = 0-100% | 88.5 (7.0) | 84.3 (6.9) | 77.2 (6.8) | 75.2 (7.0) |

*Significant differences among studies; $p < 0.05$
[a] These analyses were weighted for clustering of households from the original sample.

who reported having received mammography screening was significantly different in the four samples, with participants in the two volunteer samples reporting higher rates compared to those in Studies C and D. Perceived risk of breast cancer was also significantly different across the samples. Analyses revealed that perceived risk was higher in the two volunteer samples compared with the population-based samples ($p < 0.05$). Smoking rates were higher in the population-based samples compared with the volunteer samples, but these differences were not significant. Mental health scores differed significantly among studies, with tests indicating significance ($p < 0.05$) between Studies C and D compared with Studies A and B.

## DISCUSSION

The survey methodologies varied widely in the level of effort needed to find SMW, something not mentioned in the literature on the health of SMW. Certainly it is difficult to use probability sampling to recruit or detect relatively rare populations in sufficient numbers for a study, and high-quality sampling methods have only recently been applied to populations of diverse sexual orientation. These two reasons have driven the field of SMW research to use convenience sampling methods, such as collecting volunteers from community organizations and snowball sampling methods. However, now that the field is maturing and able to attract funding as a viable area of study (Committee on Lesbian Health Research Priorities, 1999), more scientifically appropriate and defensible methods of sampling can be used when necessary for the research question.

These more intensive and expensive population-based methods (e.g., household or individual sampling) are the only generally accepted ways to provide estimates of risk factors that are valid, that can be used to assess the risks of SMW in a specific, geographically defined area, and that can be used to provide guidance for policy decisions. Of course, even when probability sampling is used, valid inference also depends upon an acceptably high response rate. The highest yield of SMW (other than Study B) was in Study D, the area that was targeted for an enriched yield of SMW. This indicates that the method of using publicly collected data, like census data, to focus efforts to recruit a rare population might increase the yield of SMW, if such higher yield is desirable. None of these studies was designed to accurately assess the yield of SMW in the U.S., so we will have to rely on population-based surveys, like census data or well-conducted regional studies, for better estimates of sexual minority status (Blair, 1999; Blair et al., 2002; Diamant et al., 2000). Indeed, Blair and colleagues present a relatively sophisticated discussion of innovative methods of sampling clustered populations, and this method could be used in the future to sample SMW (Blair, 1999; Blair et al., 2002).

A completely plausible and appropriate alternative explanation for some of the differences between Study D and the other studies is that Study D was conducted in different geographic location from Studies A, B, and C. Therefore, we cannot conclude that any differences between Study D and the others is due to sampling method. Future research should investigate these methods of sampling exactly the same locations to make such conclusions. Despite this issue, one can speculate that area probability sampling could certainly provide better, more generalizable rates of health behaviors than simply asking for volunteers.

This comparison provides some information to use in study planning and budgeting. For example, the least expensive recruitment methods yield reasonable numbers of SMW for focused studies. This is a useful piece of knowledge, as researchers will need to estimate the number of initial contacts and likely yield to plan their studies. A recruitment procedure like the one used in Study B could be implemented with minimal resources by a research team to increase the number of SMW recruited into an ongoing study.

This study also provides guidance as to recruitment methods to use with different study designs. It is acceptable to use samples with little generalizability for certain research projects (Sudman, 1976). Participants in Studies A, B, and C agreed to participate in randomized trials of health behavior change; however, in Studies A and B, the main comparison was between the randomly selected group that received the intervention and the group that served as a control or comparison group. Generalizability is a secondary issue in randomized trials; it was certainly important but not of primary interest. The volunteer samples were very useful in recruiting relatively large numbers of women of varied sexual orientation; however, these data show that volunteer recruitment cannot be relied on for estimates of health behavior or risk factors, in that they will yield potentially inaccurate data.

The issues of differences in the values of each type of sampling can certainly begin to explain differences in rates of behaviors for SMW women, using data from the present study. Rates of current smoking, for example, were higher in the household sampling method (Study D) than the volunteer samples (Studies A and B). These differing estimates mirror the variance in published tobacco use literature (Ryan et al., 2001). Mammography screening rates differed across different studies; with the lowest rates reported by participants in the area probability sample. This indicated that we need to use probability samples to base our estimates of health behaviors. These types of estimates drive the national understanding of health disparities and are therefore important indicators of the health of a population.

These data had several limitations that limited our ability to use them fully in making cross-study comparisons. First, these studies were all framed in different ways to the participants so the recruitment rates are not strictly comparable. Women in Studies A, B, and C were recruited to a randomized trial of breast cancer risk, and participants in the two population-based studies were recruited to research health issues important to women. These differing understandings could have influenced the participation rates of both heterosexual women and SMW. There was only a limited set of variables across all four studies that were collected in a similar manner, using comparable wording and response categories. A broader grouping of variables might have yielded differing results. Study D was conducted in a separate geographical area so its results cannot be directly compared to the other studies. Finally, there are other sampling methods that might have produced different patterns of results.

In conclusion, we must pay more attention to issues of sampling in this area of research in the future. Indeed, before making health policy decisions we must conduct research using appropriate scientific methods into the health of SMW and base our considerations on these rigorously collected data.

## REFERENCES

American Association for Public Opinion Research web site. (2003). From *http:// www.aapor.org*

Andersen, M. R., & Urban, N. (1997). Physician gender and screening: Do patient differences account for differences in mammography use? *Women & Health, 26*(1), 29-39.

Blair, J. M. (1999). A probability sample of gay urban males: The use of two-phase adaptive sampling. *Journal of Sex Research, 36*(1), 39-44.

Blair, J. M., Fleming, P. L., & Karon, J. M. (2002). Trends in aids incidence and survival among racial/ethnic minority men who have sex with men, United States, 1990-1999. *Journal of Acquired Immune Deficiency Syndrome, 31*(3), 339-347.

Bowen, D. J., Burke, W., Yasui, Y., McTiernan, A., & McLerran, D. (2002). Effects of risk counseling on interest in breast cancer genetic testing for lower risk women. *Genetics in Medicine, 4*(5), 359-365.

Bowen, D. J., Powers, D., Bradford, J., McMorrow, P., Linde, R., Murphy, B. C., et al. (2004). Comparing women of differing sexual orientations using population-based sampling. *Women & Health, 40*(3), 19-34.

Bradford, J., Ryan, C., & Rothblum, E. D. (1994). National lesbian health care survey: Implications for mental health care. *Journal of Consulting and Clinical Psychology*, *62*(2), 228-242.

Burnett, C. B., Steakley, C. S., Slack, R., Roth, J., & Lerman, C. (1999). Patterns of breast cancer screening among lesbians at increased risk for breast cancer. *Women & Health*, *29*(4), 35-55.

Bybee, D., & Roeder, V. (1990). *Michigan lesbian health survey: Results relevant to aids. A report to the Michigan Organization for Human Rights and the Michigan Department of Public Health*. Lansing, Michigan: Department of Health and Human Services.

Cochran, S. D., & Mays, V. M. (1988). Disclosure of sexual preference to physicians by black lesbian and bisexual women. *The Western Journal of Medicine*, *149*(5), 616-619.

Cochran, S. D., & Mays, V. M. (2000). Relation between psychiatric syndromes and behaviorally defined sexual orientation in a sample of the US population. *American Journal of Epidemiology*, *151*(5), 516-523.

Committee on Lesbian Health Research Priorities. (1999). *Lesbian health: Current assessment and directions for the future*. Washington DC: Institute of Medicine, National Academy Press.

Deevy, S. (1990). Older lesbian women: An invisible minority. *Journal of Gerontological Nursing*, *16*(5), 35-39.

Diamant, A. L., Wold, C., Spritzer, K., & Gelberg, L. (2000). Health behaviors, health status, and access to and use of health care: A population-based study of lesbian, bisexual, and heterosexual women. *Archives of Family Medicine*, *9*(10), 1043-1051.

Ganguli, M., Lytle, M. E., Reynolds, M. D., & Dodge, H. H. (1998). Random versus volunteer selection for a community-based study. *Journal of Gerontology*, *53A*(1), m39-m46.

Hays, R. D., & Morales, L. S. (2001). The rand-36 measure of health-related quality of life. *Annals of Medicine*, *33*(5), 350-357.

Kish, L. (1965). *Survey sampling*. New York: J. Wiley.

Lehmann, J. B., Lehmann, C. U., & Kelly, P. J. (1998). Development and health care needs of lesbians. *Journal of Women's Health*, *7*(3), 379-387.

Mathews, W. C., Booth, M. W., Turner, J. D., & Kessler, L. (1986). Physicians' attitudes toward homosexuality–Survey of a california county medical society. *Western Journal of Medicine*, *144*(1), 106-110.

Meyer, H. H., & Colten, M. E. (1999). Sampling gay men: Random digit dialing versus sources in the gay community. *Journal of Homosexuality*, *37*(4), 99-110.

Polena, B., Gillispie, B., Lederman, D., & O'Hara, T. (1994). *Lesbian health care survey*. Denver, CO: Presbyterian/St.Luke's Medical Center.

Powers, D., Bowen, D., & White, J. (2001). The influence of sexual orientation on health behaviors in women. *Journal of Prevention and Intervention in the Community*, *22*(2), 43-60.

Randall, C. E. (1989). Lesbian phobia among bsn educators: A survey. *Journal of Nursing Education*, *28*(7), 302-306.

Roberts, S. J., & Sorensen, L. (1999). Health related behaviors and cancer screening of lesbians: Results from the boston lesbian health project. *Women & Health*, *28*(4), 1-12.

Ryan, H., Wortley, P. M., Easton, A., Pederson, L., & Greenwood, G. (2001). Smoking among lesbians, gays, and bisexuals: A review of the literature. *American Journal of Preventive Medicine, 21*(2), 142-149.

Sell, R. L., & Petrulio, C. (1996). Sampling homosexuals, bisexuals, gays, and lesbians for public health research: A review of the literature from 1990 to 1992. *Journal of Homosexuality, 30*(4), 31-47.

Stall, R., Mills, T. C., Williamson, J., Hart, T., Greenwood, G., Paul, J., et al. (2003). Association of co-occurring psychosocial health problems and increased vulnerability to hiv/aids among urban men who have sex with men. *Am J Public Health, 93*(6), 939-942.

Stevens, P. E., & Hall, J. M. (1988). Stigma, health beliefs and experiences with health care in lesbian women. Image: *Journal of Nursing Scholarship, 20*(2), 69-73.

Sudman, S. (1976). *Applied sampling.* New York: Academic Press.

Sudman, S. (1983). Applied sampling. In *Handbook of survey research* (pp. 145-194): Academic Press, Inc.

Trippet, S. E., & Bain, J. (1992). Reasons American lesbians fail to seek traditional health care. *Health Care for Women International, 13*(2), 145-153.

Urban, N., Taplin, S. H., Taylor, V. M., Peacock, S., Anderson, G., Conad, D., et al. (1995). Community organization to promote breast cancer screening among women ages 50-75. *Preventive Medicine, 24*(5), 477-484.

Valanis, B. G., Bowen, D. J., Bassford, T., Whitlock, E., Charney, P., & Carter, R. A. (2000). Sexual orientation and health: Comparisons in the women's health initiative sample. *Archives of Family Medicine, 9*(9), 843-853.

Warchafsky, L. (1992). *Lesbian health needs assessment.* Los Angeles: Los Angeles Gay and Lesbian Community Services Center.

Weinstein, N. D., & Klein, W. M. (1995). Resistance of personal risk perceptions to debiasing interventions. *Health Psychology, 14*(2), 132-140.

White, J. C., & Dull, V. T. (1997). Health risk factors and health-seeking behavior in lesbians. *Journal of Women's Health, 6*(1), 103-112.

doi:10.1300/J013v44n02_07

# Index

# BOOK ORDER FORM!

Order a copy of this book with this form or online at:
http://www.HaworthPress.com/store/product.asp?sku= 6002

## Preventive Health Measures
## for Lesbian and Bisexual Women

____ in softbound at $24.00 ISBN-13: 978-0-7890-3333-8 / ISBN-10: 0-7890-3333-X.
____ in hardbound at $46.00 ISBN-13: 978-0-7890-3332-1 / ISBN-10: 0-7890-3332-1.

COST OF BOOKS _____

POSTAGE & HANDLING _____
US: $4.00 for first book & $1.50
for each additional book
Outside US: $5.00 for first book
& $2.00 for each additional book.

SUBTOTAL _____
In Canada: add 6% GST. _____

STATE TAX _____
CA, IL, IN, MN, NJ, NY, OH, PA & SD residents
please add appropriate local sales tax.

FINAL TOTAL _____
If paying in Canadian funds, convert
using the current exchange rate,
UNESCO coupons welcome.

❏ BILL ME LATER:
Bill-me option is good on US/Canada/
Mexico orders only; not good to jobbers,
wholesalers, or subscription agencies.

❏ Signature _____

❏ Payment Enclosed: $_____

❏ PLEASE CHARGE TO MY CREDIT CARD:
❏ Visa ❏ MasterCard ❏ AmEx ❏ Discover
❏ Diner's Club ❏ Eurocard ❏ JCB

Account #_____

Exp Date_____

Signature_____
(Prices in US dollars and subject to change without notice.)

### PLEASE PRINT ALL INFORMATION OR ATTACH YOUR BUSINESS CARD

Name

Address

City                    State/Province                    Zip/Postal Code

Country

Tel                                    Fax

E-Mail

May we use your e-mail address for confirmations and other types of information? ❏Yes ❏No We appreciate receiving
your e-mail address. Haworth would like to e-mail special discount offers to you, as a preferred customer.
**We will never share, rent, or exchange your e-mail address.** We regard such actions as an invasion of your privacy.

Order from your **local bookstore** or directly from
**The Haworth Press, Inc.** 10 Alice Street, Binghamton, New York 13904-1580 • USA
Call our toll-free number (1-800-429-6784) / Outside US/Canada: (607) 722-5857
Fax: 1-800-895-0582 / Outside US/Canada: (607) 771-0012
E-mail your order to us: orders@HaworthPress.com
**For orders outside US and Canada,** you may wish to order through your local
sales representative, distributor, or bookseller.
For information, see http://HaworthPress.com/distributors

(Discounts are available for individual orders in US and Canada only, not booksellers/distributors.)

### Please photocopy this form for your personal use.
www.HaworthPress.com

BOF07